EMS Vehicle Operator Safety

Bob Elling, MPA, EMT-P
Editor

Robert Raheb, AS, EMT-P
Editor

National Association of Emergency Medical Technicians
Contributor

JONES & BARTLETT
LEARNING

World Headquarters
Jones & Bartlett Learning
5 Wall Street
Burlington, MA 01803
978-443-5000
info@jblearning.com
www.jblearning.com

Jones & Bartlett Learning books and products are available through most bookstores and online booksellers. To contact Jones & Bartlett Learning directly, call 800-832-0034, fax 978-443-8000, or visit our website, www.jblearning.com.

Substantial discounts on bulk quantities of Jones & Bartlett Learning publications are available to corporations, professional associations, and other qualified organizations. For details and specific discount information, contact the special sales department at Jones & Bartlett Learning via the above contact information or send an email to specialsales@jblearning.com.

10506-3

Production Credits

General Manager, Safety and Trades: Doug Kaplan
General Manager, Executive Publisher: Kimberly Brophy
VP, Product Development and Executive Editor: Christine Emerton
Acquisitions Editor—EMS and Emergency Care: Tiffany Sliter
Development Editor: Michelle Hochberg
VP, Sales, Public Safety Group: Matthew Maniscalco
Director of Sales, Public Safety Group: Patricia Einstein
Director of Ecommerce and Digital Marketing: Eric Steeves
Director of Marketing Operations: Brian Rooney

Senior Production Editor: Amanda Clerkin
VP, Manufacturing and Inventory Control: Therese Connell
Composition: Integra Software Services Pvt. Ltd.
Cover Design: Kristin E. Parker
Rights & Media Specialist: Robert Boder
Media Development Editor: Shannon Sheehan
Cover Image: © Dennis Fischer Photography/Moment Open/Getty
Printing and Binding: RR Donnelley
Cover Printing: RR Donnelley

Library of Congress Cataloging-in-Publication Data

Names: Elling, Bob, editor | Raheb, Robert, editor.
Title: EMS Vehicle Operator Safety / Bob Elling, Robert Raheb.
Description: Burlington, Massachusetts: Jones & Bartlett Learning, [2017] | Includes bibliographical references and index.
Identifiers: LCCN 2015040774 | ISBN 9780763781675
Subjects: | MESH: Ambulances. | Accidents, Traffic--prevention & control. | Automobile Driving. | Safety.
Classification: LCC TL235.8 | NLM WX 216 | DDC 362.18/8--dc23
LC record available at http://lccn.loc.gov/2015040774

6048

Printed in the United States of America
20 19 18 17 16   10 9 8 7 6 5 4 3 2 1

BRIEF CONTENTS

CONTENTS

ACKNOWLEDGMENTS

Contributors

Project Steering Committee

The following individuals were instrumental in creating the initial project proposal and shaping the scope of the course. We would like to thank them for these contributions, as well as for authoring content in the student manual.

Bob Elling, MPA, EMT-P
Clinical Instructor, Albany Medical Center/Hudson Valley
Community College Paramedic Program
CEO, High Quality Endeavors, Ltd.
Lake Placid, NY

Robert Raheb, AS, EMT-P
Lieutenant Paramedic/Certified Instructor Coordinator, FDNY
EMS (retired)
New York, NY
Simulation Training Specialist, FAAC, Inc.
Miller Place, NY

Anthony J. Deaven, EMT-P/Firefighter
Assistant Chief, Fire Aid and Safety Patrol
Lebanon, PA

Robert J. Faugh, EMT/Firefighter
Rush Fire Department
Monroe County, NY

David M. Reeves, MEd
Fire Academy Director, Guilford Technical Community College
Jamestown, NC
Captain, City Fire Department
Siler City, NC

EMS Safety Committee

Michael Szczygiel, BS
Committee Chair
Senior Loss Control Specialist, Medical Transportation
Markel Specialty Programs
Overland Park, KS

Paul Hinchey, MD
Medical Director for the EMS Safety Committee
President of East Coast Operations
Evolution Health
Dallas, TX

Taz Meyer, BS, EMT-P
Committee Co-Chair
Chief Executive Officer
St. Charles County Ambulance District
St. Peters, MO

Charlene Cobb, NRP
Community Outreach Coordinator
Sunstar Paramedics
Largo, FL

Peter Dworsky, MPH, NRP, CBRM
Corporate Director of Support Services
MONOC-Mobile Health Services
Neptune, NJ

Rob Garrett, MS, ASP, NRP
Regional Safety and Risk Manager
AMR
Greenwood Village, CO

Jason Schiederer, MS, NRP
EMS Educator
Indianapolis, IN
EPIC Implementation Director of Training
Eskenazi Health
Indianapolis, IN

National Association of Emergency Medical Technicians 2016
Board of Directors

Officers

President: Chuck Kearns
President-Elect: Dennis Rowe
Immediate Past President: Don Lundy
Secretary: Bruce Evans
Treasurer: Scott Matin
Medical Director: Paul Hinchey, MD

Directors

Sean Britton
Robert Luckritz
Chad McIntyre
Cory Richter
Aimee Binning

Jason Scheiderer
Terry David
Troy Tuke
Ben Chlapek
Matt Zavadsky

Reviewers

Daniel Armstrong, DPT, MS, EMT
Queesnsborough Community College
Bayside, NY

Mark Baisley, MA, NRP
Gold Cross Ambulance
Rochester, MN

Bruce Barry, RN, BSN, CEN, CPEN, NRP
Peak Paramedicine, LLC
Wilmington, NY

Debra L. Bell, MS, NRP
AtlantiCare Regional Medical Center EMS and Inspira Health
Network EMS
Richland, NJ

Trent R. Brass, MPH-EH, EMT-P, RRT
SwedishAmerican Health System
Rockford, IL

Dan Evans, EMT, CIC, MA, MS

Scott A. Gano, BS, NRP, FP-C, CCEMTP
Columbus State Community College
Columbus, OH

Greg P. Henington, NRP, LP
Chief
Terlingua Fire & EMS, Inc.
Terlingua, TX

Ed Hollowell, RN, CFRN, CEN, NRP, CCP-C, FF
Regional Fire & Rescue
Avondale, AZ

Scott A. Jaeggi, BA, EMT-P
Instructor
Rio Hondo College Fire Academy
Santa Fe Springs, CA

K. C. Jones, NRP, NCEE
Associate Professor
North Arkansas College
Harrison, AR

Rich Kaufman, MBA, NRP
EMS Institute
Pittsburgh, PA

Sgt. Charles Kean, MA, EMT-P
Springfield Police Department Emergency Response Team
Lincoln Land Community College
Springfield, IL

Melodie J. Kolmetz, MPAS, PA-C, EMT-P
Monroe Community College
Rochester, NY

Daniel W. Lewis, MBA, NRP
Indianapolis EMS
Indianapolis, IN

Michael E. Lisa, BS
NJ EMT/Instructor, Fire Officer (retired)
Trinitas Medical Center EMS Training
Elizabeth, NJ

Los Alamos Fire Department
Los Alamos, NM

Susan M. Macklin, BS, AAS, NC Paramedic
Central Carolina Community College
Olivia, NC

Jeanette S. Mann, RN, BSN, NRP
Director of Emergency Medical Services Program
Dabney S. Lancaster Community College
Clifton Forge, VA

Donna McHenry, MS, NRP
University of New Mexico
Albuquerque, NM

Scott Miller
EMS Program Director
San Jose City College
San Jose, CA

Keith Noble, MS, LP, NRP
Commander
Austin-Travis County EMS
Austin, TX

Chris Ottolini, EMT-P, CPT
Paramedic Supervisor, Coast Life Support District
Gualala, CA
Adjunct Instructor, Santa Rosa Junior College Public Safety Training Center
Windsor, CA

Allen O. Patterson, NRP, LP, CCP, EMSC
Advance Coordinator
Lamar State College-Orange
Houston, TX

Paul Richardson, EMT-P
Hancock County EMS
Carthage, IL

Nicholas Russell, AAS, NRP, EMS-I, FI-3
Edgewood Fire/EMS
Edgewood, KY

T. Troy Salazar, BS, OM; NRP; AZ, CO, NM Paramedic
Southwest Colorado Community College
Durango, CO

Jared C. Schoenfeld, CCEMTP, PNCCT, NRP
Regional Transport Service
Mission Hospital
Asheville, NC

Bradley L. Spratt, MEd, LP, CSP
Northwest Technical Solutions
Katy, TX

Robert Stakem, BS, CCEMTP, NCEE
Harrisburg Area Community College
Harrisburg, PA

Daniel A. Svenson, BA, RN, NRP
Portland Fire Department
Portland, ME

Sara VanDusseldorp, NRP, CCEMTP, NCEE
North Lake County EMS
Waukegan, IL

Gary S. Walter, MS, NRP, EMSI
International Rescue & Relief, Union College
Lincoln, NE

Roger G. Wootten, BS, NRP
Northeast Alabama Community College
Rainsville, AL

Photoshoot Acknowledgments

We would like to thank the following individuals and institutions for their collaboration on the photoshoots for this project. Their assistance was greatly appreciated.

Barry Bashkoff
Cromwell Emergency Vehicles, Inc.
Clifton Park, NY

Anthony M. Caliguire, NRP, CIC
Paramedic Instructor Coordinator, HVCC Paramedic Program
Troy, NY
Lieutenant Paramedic, Scotia Fire Department
Scotia, NY

Adam Henery
Scotia Fire Department
Scotia, NY

Danielle Matteo
Bay Shore-Brightwaters Rescue Ambulance, Inc.
Bay Shore, NY

Doug Ruso, EMT
Albany, NY

Bay Shore-Brightwaters Rescue Ambulance, Inc.
Bay Shore, NY

Hudson Valley Community College
Troy, NY

Scotia Fire Department
Scotia, NY

PREFACE

Thousands of EMS vehicle crashes occur each year, which suggests a clear training gap that needs to be filled. Dedicated to continually improving EMS education, the editors of and contributors to EMS Vehicle Operator Safety (EVOS) have used their collective knowledge and breadth of experience both in the field and in the classroom to design a robust and engaging EMS vehicle operator training course. Developed in partnership with the National Association of Emergency Medical Technicians (NAEMT), EVOS is a national program with an open format that allows jurisdictions and agencies to incorporate local laws and regulations and standard operating procedures (SOPs), making it a course that is credible, flexible, and relevant to all EMS providers.

Why *EVOS?*

Course Aims

EVOS focuses on what matters most—creating and maintaining a culture of safety. Its paramount goal is to reduce crashes, injuries, and fatalities involving EMS vehicles and providers. Built on the most current research, this evidence-based course underscores that both vehicle dynamics and human factors contribute to collisions, and that certain behaviors must be changed in order to promote a culture of safe driving. It emphasizes increasing the emergency vehicle operator's awareness and understanding of vehicle safety, and the critical importance of understanding local laws and SOPs. It challenges EMS providers to think critically by analyzing real-life scenarios and typical crashes, highlighting the specific hazards that lead to collisions and offering practical strategies to avoid them.

Course Education Philosophy

The EVOS course philosophy is rooted in the belief that analyzing actual crashes offers invaluable lessons that can be applied to future vehicle operator training and behavior. It is essential to take the time to share best practices and the hard lessons learned from past errors so that others will not repeat them.

Vehicle collisions are *not* accidents. In fact, the National Safety Council refers to them as *preventable crashes*. EVOS firmly refrains from using the term *motor vehicle accident* because conscious choices and behaviors lead to collisions; they do not simply happen.

Enhancing EMS Vehicle Operator Training

EVOS was designed and developed by a team of seasoned field practitioners and educators with a wealth of unique experience in EMS safety and vehicle operator training.

- Bob Elling has dedicated much of his career to attempting to quantify the ambulance crash problem and remediate it through policy and education changes. As a Training Coordinator with New York State EMS, he helped develop seatbelt use policies and piloted a New York State–sponsored Emergency Vehicle Operator Course (EVOC) instructor course. He also published one of the first articles in the *Journal of Emergency Medical Services (JEMS)* on the topic of ambulance crashes and developed the Ambulance Accident Prevention Seminar, which was rolled out as a continuing education workshop and taught to over 20,000 EMTs.
- Rob Raheb observed early in his EMS career that there were no standard criteria for driving emergency vehicles. When he became the lieutenant in charge of the New York City Fire Department Bureau of EMS (FDNY EMS) emergency vehicle operator course years later, he sought to enhance it by researching and studying the science and art of driving and becoming both an Accident Investigator and a New York State–certified EVOC instructor. He later developed a driving simulator program and, after conducting an 8-year study to explore its effectiveness, demonstrated that by providing participants with opportunities to build their judgment and decision-making skills, simulation training could offer immense value. Today Rob travels around the country teaching emergency vehicle operator training and promoting simulation training.
- EVOS was developed in partnership with the NAEMT, as an initiative to expand the culture of EMS safety portrayed in the organization's EMS Safety course into a new program that addresses the emergency vehicle operator's specific needs. The NAEMT's EMS Safety Committee played a critical role by reviewing the EVOS course materials to ensure their alignment with current guidelines and the techniques and best practices of the EMS Safety curriculum. Key contributions to the course's scope and content were made by

two members in particular: Charlene Cobb and Jason Scheiderer. Charlene has been a contributing member of the EMS Safety Foundation since 2007, and has held positions of EVOC Instructor and Education Coordinator, among others. Jason Scheiderer is a certified Indiana EVOC Instructor and an NAEMT EMS Safety Instructor.

The editors of and contributors to EVOS sincerely hope that you will find the course a valuable part of your EMS education.

National Association of Emergency Medical Technicians

The National Association of Emergency Medical Technicians (NAEMT) was founded in 1975 to serve and represent the professional interests of EMS practitioners, including paramedics, emergency medical technicians, and emergency medical responders. NAEMT members work in all sectors of EMS, including government service agencies, fire departments, hospital-based ambulance services, private companies, industrial and special operations settings, and the military.

One of NAEMT's principal activities is EMS continuing education. The mission of NAEMT continuing education programs is to improve patient care through high-quality, cost-effective, evidence-based education that strengthens and enhances the knowledge and skills of EMS practitioners.

NAEMT strives to provide the highest quality continuing education programs. All NAEMT continuing education program are developed by highly experienced EMS educators, clinicians, and medical directors. Course content incorporates the latest research, newest techniques, and innovative approaches in EMS learning. All NAEMT continuing education programs promote critical thinking as the foundation for providing quality care. This is based on the belief that EMS practitioners make the best decisions on behalf of their patients when given a sound foundation of evidence-based knowledge and key principles.

Once developed, continuing education programs are tested and refined to ensure that course materials are clear, accurate, and relevant to the needs of EMS practitioners. Finally, all continuing education programs are regularly updated no less than every 4 years to ensure that the content incorporates the most up-to-date research and practices.

NAEMT provides ongoing support to its instructors and the EMS training sites that hold its courses. Over 1,800 training sites, including colleges, EMS agencies, hospitals, and other training centers located in the United States and over 50 other countries, offer NAEMT continuing education programs. NAEMT headquarters staff work with the network of continuing education program volunteers from committee members; national, regional, and state coordinators; and affiliate faculty to provide administrative and educational support.

CHAPTER 1

Introduction to EMS Vehicle Operator Safety

OBJECTIVES

1.1 Outline the history of emergency vehicle operator training.

1.2 Explain the need for an emergency medical services (EMS) vehicle operator course.

1.3 Discuss the profile of a typical EMS vehicle crash.

1.4 Explain the goals of the EMS Vehicle Operator Safety (EVOS) course.

1.5 Describe the emergency vehicle operator selection process.

1.6 Explain the value of analyzing cases of EMS vehicle crashes.

SCENARIO

You picked up an extra midnight shift at your part-time medic job in Queens, New York. Tomorrow is your day off at your regular medic job in Manhattan so you can go home and sleep in the morning. Since midnight, it has been quiet, and you are on only your second call. It is 3:00 AM and you and your partner, Pete, are transporting a 72-year-old woman to the hospital. She had a chief complaint of chest pain with a long cardiac history, so you have her resting in a semi-Fowler's position on your stretcher as you head to the emergency department (ED). You have already done an assessment and are following the STEMI protocol and have transmitted the 12-lead ECG to the ED. After administering care, you turn to some light conversation about her grandchildren to calm her down. Your partner is driving with the emergency lights on but traveling within the speed limit because there is very little traffic on the street at this time. He is wearing a seatbelt because your service's policies and procedures require it, and you both know that it is good common sense. You are seated on the crew bench, and the life-pack monitor is sitting on the bench next to you. Both you and the device are not restrained, which is both legal and within the department policies.

As your partner proceeds through an intersection where he has the green light, another vehicle traveling at a high rate of speed runs the red light and the ambulance strikes the vehicle's left front quarter panel. In the moment when your partner sees the vehicle coming, he attempts to stop the ambulance and reaches for the brake as he screams, "Hold on!" Sitting in the patient compartment and in the middle of a conversation with the patient, you do not see any of the warning signs that the ambulance is about to collide with another vehicle. You and the patient are simply taken by surprise. The patient, who was restrained, is shaken up a bit, but, fortunately, she did not leave the stretcher. You were not restrained and had nothing to grab to steady yourself. You were thrown forward into the well between the driver's compartment and the patient compartment of this Type 3 ambulance. Everything happened so quickly. In an instant, you struck your head and were knocked unconscious; you did not see the airborne, 17.5-pound ECG monitor or feel it strike you in the lumbar spine. Fortunately, your partner was not rendered unconscious and responded quickly by bringing the vehicle to a stop before it hit a utility pole. His first act is to call for the police and two additional ambulances. Before he has a chance to get out and check on you, the other driver speeds away.

As you regain consciousness, you hear a lot of commotion. A crew is moving the elderly patient to another ambulance. She was shaken up a little, but has not sustained any new injuries. You later learn that she was admitted to the critical care unit to be monitored on telemetry for the night. Although your ambulance was totaled, your partner experienced only some neck strain and minor glass cuts. After several hours, the police finally locate the drunk driver who crashed into your ambulance; he was driving with a suspended license. He has no injuries.

Your injuries include a broken thumb, a concussion, and two small fractures in your lumbar spine with no neurologic deficits. The back injury will result in a couple of weeks of light duty and a lifetime of intermittent back problems. All things considered, you feel lucky that this crash did not end your career. After some reflection, you realize that you learned a lesson you can share with other EMS providers for the rest of your career: Always be prepared for a collision by securing all equipment, and be sure you are always belted in during transport while in the patient compartment of the ambulance.

1. What were the preventable factors that led to this collision?
2. What factors were you unable to control that led to this collision?
3. Could the outcome have been the same had this scenario not involved a collision with another vehicle?

Brief History of Emergency Vehicle Operator Training

It has been well documented that emergency medical services (EMS) vehicle collisions cause significant injury, death, and property damage each year in the United States. In one analysis by the **National Highway Traffic Safety Administration (NHTSA)** of a 10-year period (1991–2000), there were 301,404 emergency vehicles involved in nonfatal collisions and 1,565 crashes involving fatalities. Over the years, a number of training programs have been developed with the goal of better educating drivers of emergency vehicles in an effort to dramatically reduce the number of tragic accidents. The number one rule of medicine has always been, "First, do no harm." Yet, each year across the United States, patients, bystanders, family members, and EMS providers are killed or seriously injured during collisions involving ambulances. These collisions, injuries, and deaths do not discriminate based on response variables: volunteer or paid staff, private or public agency, 9-1-1 response or interfacility transfer. These tragedies can no longer be brushed under the rug and hidden from the public view for the insurance companies and lawyers to fight about. Today, the Internet nearly guarantees that moments after a collision occurs details will reach the news media, social media sites, and trade journal websites, and the entire country will become aware of the incident.

One of the first efforts to address the lack of standardized education for emergency vehicle operators was the U.S. Department of Transportation's (DOT's) development of the Emergency Vehicle Operator Course (EVOC). The original 1978 course was general and designed to reduce the incidence of emergency vehicle collisions, so it included sections for police, fire, and EMS vehicles. The 1978 edition of EVOC was revised in 1995 to the *Emergency Vehicle Operator Course (Ambulance): National Standard Curriculum.* The revised curriculum addresse emergency vehicle operations as they relate to the operation of ambulances, and includes didactic and skills range components. There were some limitations and mixed opinions of EVOC. Some services did not believe they had the space or instructors to teach the program. Other services have had success integrating EVOC into their on-the-job training of new employees and retraining of those who were involved in a collision.

With such mixed opinions of EVOC, other programs were developed, such as the following:

1. Coaching the Emergency Vehicle Operator (CEVO) courses were first introduced in the early 1990s for ambulance, fire, and police personnel and have been presented to over 500,000 emergency professionals.
2. The Ambulance Accident Prevention Seminar (AAPS) was developed in 1989 by New York State EMS Program staff under a Governor's Traffic Safety grant. This 1-day program was designed to be an attitude adjustment and awareness program, presenting information on driving laws and common causes of ambulance crashes. There was no skills component to the program, but nearly 25,000 providers were trained in just a few years.
3. The Volunteer Firemen's Insurance Services (VFIS), through its Emergency Vehicle Driver Training program, has partnered with fire and EMS leaders for more than 30 years to enable the continuing development of policy and program enhancements, specialized education, and consulting for management needs. VFIS is committed to protecting the resources of emergency service organizations and promoting the health and interest of its members.
4. Many services have developed their own versions of EVOC based on standards from the Occupational Safety and Health Administration (OSHA), National Fire Protection Association (NFPA), and their respective states.

In addition to the available courses to train the emergency vehicle operator, the guidelines or objectives for driver training have been discussed in a number of NFPA standards as well as the 2009 *National EMS Education Standards.* There also are a few near-miss websites where reports of crashes or close calls are discussed so that others can avoid making similar mistakes.

Estimates of the Depth and Breadth of the Problem

In a review of New York State (NYS) ambulance crash data (courtesy of the NYS Department of Motor Vehicles), some interesting data were revealed. Based on 28 years of NYS data, there were 9,599 ambulance collisions—an average of 343 per year. During this time, 78 persons were killed (an average of 3 per year) and 13,701 persons injured (an average of 489 per year). The profile of a typical crash during this time includes clear weather, daylight hours, a right-angle lateral collision, a dry road surface, and an intersection that had a traffic control device.

These data reveal similar trends analyzed over an 18-year period in NYS, serving as the basis for the article titled "Dispelling Myths on Ambulance Accidents" published in the *Journal of Emergency Medical Services* in July of 1989. The data seem to repeat the same story, even after 10 more years of data have been added to the database.

Human Behaviors

If you saw a paramedic starting an IV without wearing gloves, you would certainly notice the error and quickly point it out; however, you would not have felt the same concern in the 1970s. How was that mindset changed?

Ambulance design is constantly changing to improve safety, yet these vehicles are still dangerous to their occupants. The fact is, no matter how sound the design, construction, and mechanics of an ambulance, it will always be used in a fundamentally unpredictable pursuit. It will be used to negotiate traffic (which is itself unpredictable) in an urgent manner while trying to obtain the right of way. It will be used to transport individuals, sometimes engaged in a desperate fight for survival, and their medical providers, who despite their skill and attention to safety protocols will sometimes feel less inclined to worry about their own safety than the needs of their patients. EMS providers may disregard measures such as restraining themselves or their equipment in order to save seconds while working on patients; this can be a deadly choice. Just like their patients, EMS providers in the patient compartment of an ambulance are subject to all the laws of physics should a collision occur.

In addressing transport safety, the questions must not focus solely on vehicle dynamics but must consider also human dynamics. For example, what human behaviors need to be changed for operators of the ambulance? Should administrators limit the number of consecutive hours EMS providers can work without a sleep break?

New Jersey has passed Maggie's Law (effective August 2003), which makes it possible for a drowsy driver who accidentally kills someone to be charged with vehicle homicide (up to 10 years in prison and a fine of $100,000). In the NHTSA 2002 survey on driver distractions (National Survey of Distracted and Drowsy Driving Attitudes and Behavior: 2002), the average drowsy driving experience is associated with the following characteristics:

- The driver averaged 6 hours of sleep the previous night (24% had slept fewer than 5 hours).
- The driver had been driving for an average of 2.9 hours (22% had been driving for more than 4 hours).
- The collision occurred while driving on an interstate-type highway with posted speeds of 55 mph or higher (59%).
- Nearly half (48%) of drivers nodded off between 9:00 PM and 6:00 AM.

Why is this human behavior not changing? This course, EMS Vehicle Operator Safety (EVOS), focuses on this question and the following related questions:

- Do EMS agencies share best practices, such as policies, training programs, and public education, and learn from mistakes?
- Do services conduct motor vehicle record reviews on all ambulance operators?
- How much of a factor is the "hero mentality"—rushing to save seconds? Many EMS providers fall prey to the belief that arriving at the scene or the hospital 30 seconds earlier would make a difference in patient outcome, although it rarely does.
- Does better use of emergency medical dispatch protocols help reduce the number of emergency (lights and sirens) responses? Jeff Clawson, MD, considered the "Father of Medical Priority Dispatch," thinks so.
- Is everyone really a good and safe driver? Is there a place in EMS for the poor drivers?
- Are crashes an acceptable part of doing business?
- Is road rage increasing?
- Are there best practices for use of sirens and warning devices?

Some Concerns and Some Progress

As research into ambulance design and responses grows, there will be better science to guide the construction of new units. Better designs coupled with changes in attitudes and behaviors should reduce ambulance crashes and associated morbidity and mortality. The Centers for Disease Control and Prevention (CDC) has begun to review the data on injuries to EMS workers. Recognizing that there is a problem is a good first step. Their research raises a number of critical questions; for example, it is no longer considered acceptable to drive the ambulance while intoxicated, but what about over-the-counter (OTC) medication use or driving while drowsy?

In addition to organizations like the CDC turning their attention to the problem of EMS driving safety, the legal community, insurance companies, and OSHA are all getting involved and generating more conversation about the issue.

Certainly the data available on EMS-related crashes are disconcerting, even now when providers are more conscious of safety than ever before.

The Emergency Vehicle Operator Selection Process

A key question in the emergency vehicle operator selection process is, are we selecting only a driver or are we selecting EMTs and paramedics and training them as drivers? The latter scenario is more common. Human resources departments provide selection criteria that should be developed with plenty of input from the EMS personnel.

There are few legal restrictions on becoming an emergency vehicle operator; these regulations are state imposed. Unlike other professional vehicle operators, such as bus or truck drivers, whose requirements include formal training, an evaluation process to demonstrate competency, and a physical exam, the emergency vehicle operator's minimum requirements include age and a valid driver's license. This means that the conversation of how to keep risky or unskilled emergency vehicle operators out of the driver's seat falls to individual services.

There should be focused discussions about the qualities that make a good emergency vehicle operator and should undoubtedly include such concerns as background motor vehicle operator checks, maturity, responsibility, and intrinsic motivation. Most states have a process for the department to obtain an abstract of the prospective emergency vehicle operator's driving record. History can be an important predictor of future behavior, and not hiring someone with a history of driving problems is important. It is also important to create a culture of safe driving in every service, in which dangerous driving and risky behaviors are unacceptable and reporting such behaviors is encouraged.

Lessons Learned From Actual Crashes

Most crashes are reviewed by one or many agencies to determine the factors that caused the crash and ways it could have been prevented. At a minimum, the local police department and your EMS agency should investigate all crashes. At some point, once the legal dust settles, there should be a report that can be reviewed. If there is a lawsuit or the potential for one, it might be difficult to obtain copies of materials to analyze. In some instances, there may have been oversight review from an outside agency, insurance investigators, the state health department, the state or local police, the National Traffic Safety Board, and other parties, which can produce very useful reports to review and formulate, from a quality improvement perspective, the lessons we should all learn from the incident.

This manual presents 18 scenarios, which have all been developed from actual crashes. This is just a starting point. The extent of the problem should become clear to you as you seriously consider the factors—mostly human factors—which led to these collisions. Some cutting-edge leaders in the EMS industry have taken the lessons learned from analyzing crashes and moved them into simulations so more providers can benefit from them.

There is tremendous value in moving these lessons into simulations to help providers avoid similar mistakes. Typically, simulations have been most useful in high-risk or high-price incidents, which happen in low frequency. In respect to driving an emergency vehicle, which is a high-frequency activity with a perceived low risk, EMS needs to move away from the perception that simulation teaches how to drive, toward the understanding that simulation can be used to help avoid replicating choices that led to the crash itself. In that way, the simulation is actually being used to prevent low-frequency, high-risk, or costly events. The airline industry has extensive experience with simulations, which have helped to move the fatality incidence from one per million miles to one per billion miles traveled. Today, simulation is not only considered acceptable flight training, but it also accounts for more hours of training than actual flight time. Captain Sullenberger, who was presented with a sudden in-flight emergency, had to safely glide US Airways Flight 1549 to a landing on the Hudson River in New York City FIGURE 1-1 . He attributed his success, and that of his crew, to the extensive training they had received, particularly flight simulatons.

The military also employs simulations in their training of medics, utilizing high-fidelity mannequins as well as portable computer simulations. The entire military model of training was reviewed and revised extensively in response to the famous Black Hawk Down incident, in which over 100 Army Rangers were ambushed and entrapped by hundreds of heavily armed Somalis. During this incident, a soldier treated by the medics bled to death from his injuries. In after-action review of the incident, the leaders promised that nothing like this would ever happen again, and thus, the medical training of all soldiers has been updated.

Figure 1-1   On January 15, 2009, Captain Chesley Burnett Sullenberger III successfully landed US airways flight 1549 in the Hudson River off Manhattan, NY.
© Steven Day/AP Photo.

The EMS industry has moved slowly into simulations, particularly for driver training. Simulations are discussed in greater detail in Chapter 11.

SAFETY POINTER

The best way to save time getting to the call location is to know your district well and take a moment to look up the location on the map and/or review the GPS driving route before heading out to the call. Simply leaving the station without a clear idea of the call location puts extra stress on the emergency vehicle operator and can create a distraction while operating the vehicle.

WRAP-UP

Summary

- There have been, and continue to be, too many ambulance crashes in the United States resulting in injuries and fatalities.
- The Emergency Vehicle Operator Course was the first national effort to improve emergency vehicle operator education. Other programs have since joined it in the effort to reduce EMS vehicle crashes.
- The human behaviors that contribute to collisions and fatalities must be identified and changed.
- This course, EMS Vehicle Operator Safety (EVOS), presents sample policies and discussions of actual crashes so that we can all learn from these tragedies.
- An important part of the development of emergency vehicle operators is the selection and education process.

Glossary

Centers for Disease Control and Prevention (CDC) The government agency that works to protect American health, safety, and security from all types of diseases, including those caused by human error and preventable problems.

emergency vehicle operator The individual driving the emergency vehicle, generally an ambulance, who has the ability to operate it in the emergency mode (activating the lights and/or sirens).

Emergency Vehicle Operator Course (EVOC) A course launched in 1978 by the U.S. Department of Transportation to reduce the incidence of emergency vehicle collisions.

National Fire Protection Association (NFPA) A standards-setting entity that develops gold standards for the fire service.

National Highway Traffic Safety Administration (NHTSA) An agency of the U.S. Department of Transportation responsible for ensuring safe driving conditions.

CHAPTER 2

Making Safety a Priority

OBJECTIVES

2.1 Discuss the importance of safety in any emergency response.

2.2 Discuss the importance of ensuring mental preparedness by avoiding or managing sleep deprivation, excessive emotion, stress, and any physical ailments that may inhibit decision making.

2.3 Discuss the importance of developing a "safety-first" attitude.

2.4 Discuss the importance of proper seatbelt placement, airbags, headrest positioning, mirror position, the use of a spotter, and equipment restraint.

2.5 Explain how to secure a patient to the stretcher.

2.6 Demonstrate how to safely transport adult and child patients and passengers.

2.7 Demonstrate how to establish a safe work zone in the event of a roadway incident.

2.8 Outline the appropriate steps to respond safely to mechanical failure.

SCENARIO

On July 13, 2001, a 27-year-old female EMT died when the ambulance she was working in struck a support column for an elevated train track. The EMT had been riding unrestrained in the patient compartment while attending to a patient during a nonemergency medical transport. Since the transport was a nonemergency it is not clear whether being unrestrained was necessary to patient care.

Leading up to the collision, the crew departed the hospital with the patient at 11:56 AM. The patient had been placed supine on the cot, secured with lap-belt-type leg and hip restraints and loaded into the ambulance. The ambulance was traveling southbound without lights and siren on a two-lane city street. At approximately 12:15 PM, 1.5 miles from the hospital, the driver drifted through the northbound lane toward oncoming traffic and struck an elevated train track support column at an estimated speed of 26 mph FIGURE 2-1 and FIGURE 2-2 . At approximately 12:20 PM, the EMT/driver called the office of the ambulance service to report the incident. At about the same time, witnesses called 9-1-1.

Figure 2-1 Overhead view of the crash scene.
© Jones & Bartlett Learning.

Figure 2-2 The front/driver's side view of the damage that resulted from the ambulance striking the track support column ("El" pillar).
Courtesy of Rob Raheb.

During the collision, the patient was partially ejected from the cot restraints and struck the rear-facing captain's seat at the front of the patient compartment. The EMT/driver, who was riding unrestrained, contacted the vehicle's dash and the inflating airbag. The EMT attending to the patient impacted and broke a handrail at the end of the squad bench and struck a cabinet at the front of the patient compartment.

The EMT/driver, EMT, and patient were transported by ambulance to a hospital. The EMT from the patient compartment was pronounced dead as a result of injuries, including a thoracic spine cord laceration, complete cord syndrome with dislocation, bilateral lung contusions, and cerebellum subarachnoid hemorrhage.

A conclusive determination could not be made as to why the ambulance veered left across traffic and struck the support column. However, the National Automotive Sampling System (NASS) case file for this incident indicated that no avoidance maneuvers had been attempted and listed "inattentive or distracted, sleepy or fell asleep" under the category for distraction. Witnesses interviewed said that the driver admitted having no recollection of the crash.

1. Have you ever caught yourself drifting off while driving your personal vehicle or the ambulance?
2. How often do you use all available restraints for yourself and your patient?
3. Have you ever had a close call because you were not focused while driving?

Sources: Centers for Disease Control and Prevention. (2003). Ambulance crash-related injuries among emergency medical services workers—United States, 1991–2002. *Morbidity and Mortality Weekly Report, 52*(8), 154–156. Retrieved from http://www.cdc.gov/mmwr/preview/mmwrhtml/mm5208a3.htm; Centers for Disease Control and Prevention. (2004). Emergency medical technician dies in ambulance crash—New York. Fatality Assessment and Control Evaluation (FACE) Program. *National Institute for Occupational Safety and Health (NIOSH) In-house FACE Report.* Retrieved from http://www.cdc.gov/niosh/face/In-house/full200112.html.

Introduction

An EMS provider's abilities, skills, and knowledge of emergency vehicle operation contribute to every EMS response. Every year there are millions of EMS responses that place the EMS provider and the general public at risk. The priority for every EMS provider is to ensure his or her own safety and the safety of his or her partner, the patient, and any passengers. Your own personal safety must be placed ahead of everyone else's. Ensuring your own safety includes being mentally and physically prepared, fastening your seatbelt, and making sure the unit is safe to operate.

You play a key role in keeping your partner safe by ensuring the proper use of seatbelts, in both the front and the patient compartments of the ambulance. Proper safety belts are also important for patient safety, including all of the gurney shoulder straps provided by the manufacturer. The best patient care can be provided only by enforcing a "safety-first" attitude and ensuring that everyone around does the same. The right thing to do may feel uncomfortable, such as telling your partner to put on a seatbelt before you move the vehicle or asking the driver to slow down. However, vehicle collisions continue to be the main cause of death for EMS providers (aeromedical excluded), and it is important to do the right thing: Practice safety first, all the time.

Personal Preparedness

As the operator of an emergency vehicle, you are responsible for safe vehicle operation, including the safety of the public and those in the vehicle. Emergency vehicle operators must be both mentally and physically prepared to perform their jobs. Mental preparation includes an awareness and management of sleep deprivation, emotions, and stress while maintaining physical awareness and a safety-first attitude.

Sleep Deprivation

Sleep deprivation is a common cause of driver error. Most adults require 7 to 9 hours of sleep per night. Being well rested improves concentration, reaction times, and physical capabilities. Drowsy driving occurs when a person does not get the proper amount of sleep. Common signs of drowsy driving include:

- Difficulty focusing, frequent blinking, or heavy eyelids
- Daydreaming; wandering or disconnected thoughts
- Microsleeping
- Trouble remembering the last few miles driven; missing exits or traffic signs
- Yawning repeatedly or rubbing your eyes
- Trouble keeping your head up
- Drifting from your lane, tailgating, or hitting a shoulder rumble strip
- Feeling restless and irritable

It is your personal responsibility to ensure that you are well rested for your shift and are not a danger to yourself or others.

According to the National Sleep Foundation's (NSF) 2009 Sleep in America poll, 54% of respondents indicated that they had driven a vehicle within the past year while feeling drowsy; 28% of those who drive reported having actually fallen asleep at the wheel. The National Highway Traffic Safety Administration (NHTSA) estimates that about 100,000 police-reported crashes are the direct result of driver fatigue annually. International estimates fault drowsy driving for 10% to 30% of all automobile crashes. The NHTSA and the Centers for Disease Control and Prevention report that 2.5% of all fatal crashes are a result of drowsy driving, which results in an estimated 1,550 deaths each year. Drowsy driving annually results in an estimated 2% of all injury crashes or 71,000 injuries. These large numbers result in an estimated $12.5 billion in monetary losses annually. Unfortunately, these figures are believed to be low estimates and may not capture the true prevalence of drowsy driving-rated incidents, since without a way to test for it, it is difficult to attribute crashes to sleepiness.

According to the NSF's 2001 Sleep in America poll, a number of the nearly three-quarters of U.S. adults (71%) who drive a car to and from work are drowsy drivers. More than one-quarter of those surveyed (27%) reported they had driven drowsy to or from work at least a few days a month, 12% said they drove drowsy a few days a week, and 4% reported they drove drowsy every day or almost every day. Drowsy drivers are more likely to have lapses of attention while on the road.

Sleep deprivation and fatigue may also affect behaviors that can lead to crashes, such as speeding. According to the NSF's 2000 Sleep in America poll, when asked about their behavior while driving drowsy, 42% of respondents said they become stressed, 32% said they get impatient, and 12% reported that they tend to drive faster.

The NSF also notes several trends about drivers who fall asleep at the wheel. Drivers are more likely to fall asleep on high-speed, long, boring, rural highways. However, those who live in urban areas are more likely to doze off while driving compared to rural or suburban counterparts (24% vs. 17%). Crashes or near misses most commonly occur between the hours of 4:00 AM and 6:00 AM, 12:00 AM and 2:00 AM, or 2:00 PM and 4:00 PM. According to the NSF's 2005 Sleep in America poll, of the approximately one-third of drivers who reported having ever fallen asleep, or microslept, while driving, 13% reported having done so at least once a month. Nearly one-quarter of adults say they know someone personally who has crashed due to falling asleep at the wheel.

Drowsy driving has been compared to another extremely dangerous and illegal practice: driving under the influence of alcohol. In the United States, 0.08% blood alcohol concentration is considered impaired and illegal. There are studies that show that being awake for 18 consecutive hours is impairment equal to a blood alcohol concentration of 0.05%. Being awake for a full 24 hours produced impairment similar to a 0.096% blood alcohol concentration, which is legally intoxicated in all 50 states.

Wrecks from drowsy driving can result in high personal and economic costs. Several drowsy driving incidents have resulted in jail sentences for the driver. These crashes have resulted in multimillion-dollar settlements against drivers and their companies.

These costs do not include the damage to reputation and accompanying losses that a company will have due to news of the crash.

As an emergency vehicle operator, you are ultimately responsible for the safe operation of the vehicle. However, companies should take precautions and create policies that ensure providers have the opportunity to rest before shifts. This should include mandating time off between shifts and setting maximum consecutive hours of work to prevent impairment. EMS is currently one of the very few transportation-related fields that is not regulated with mandatory time off and rest periods.

SAFETY POINTER

It is your responsibility as an EMS provider to ensure you are well rested, having received a recommended 7–9 hours of sleep, and fit for duty prior to the start of your shift.

Emotions

Although emotions can be difficult to manage, EMS providers have a responsibility to be emotionally prepared for their shifts by not bringing personal distractions to work or allowing professional challenges to affect decision-making abilities. Some common emotions that can affect your ability to make decisions are anger, love, hate, fear, grief, and happiness.

Loss of control of emotions can interfere with the ability to think and focus. This lack of focus and inability to concentrate create an environment in which a driver can be distracted, affecting the ability to process information and increasing risk-taking behavior. As part of your personal preparedness, it is your responsibility to ensure that you are emotionally capable of operating an emergency vehicle. The type of run, the patient, the behavior of other drivers, and many other factors can be triggers for cumulative stress reactions. The emergency vehicle operator needs to be able to recognize and control those reactions when driving.

Stress

EMS providers are constantly placed in high-stress environments. You must be able to properly manage your stress level and prevent it from interfering with your decision-making abilities. Stress associated with an EMS response can occur frequently and affects each individual differently. For example, your stress may increase when a call involves a pediatric patient, while another person's stress may increase when the call involves an Alzheimer's patient. These responses may be delayed or cumulative, manifesting in reaction to other situations.

As stress levels increase, so do levels of adrenaline and cortisone, as the body prepares for a fight-or-flight response. The increase in these stress hormones affects the vehicle operator by increasing pulse rate and elevating blood pressure. Adrenaline also causes the pupils to dilate and take in more light, increasing the field of vision.

However, as blood is redistributed from certain areas of the brain to the muscles and internal organs, peripheral vision is decreased (tunnel vision), which consequently narrows the visual field. Increased levels of stress hormones may also result in increased risky behavior and more emotional reactions, such as frustration or anger. In addition to the physical effects of adrenaline and cortisone, stress may also affect a person physically, causing gastrointestinal discomfort, headaches, or back pain. Longer-term and consistent exposure to stress can lead to memory and concentration problems, which are the enemy of the emergency vehicle operator.

At one time or another, all EMS providers will be adversely affected by job-related stress. It is imperative that EMS providers recognize stress and change their behaviors to compensate for its adverse effects. An excellent way to combat the effects of stress is to practice safe driving habits every day. During stressful events, people who have reinforced good habits with education and training are able to make better decisions. By practicing safe vehicle operations every day, you will reduce your risk during a stressful event. The key is to stay focused, understand that other drivers will react to the presence of your emergency vehicle in a variety of ways, and remain prepared and in control when other drivers undertake crazy maneuvers. Maintaining self-control involves not internalizing others' actions and creating a new stressor.

Physical Awareness

Your state of health, both physical and mental, can affect your ability to operate an emergency vehicle. Therefore, physical awareness is an important part of ensuring your preparedness and safety. Physical awareness includes being sensitive to any health problems. It is also important to remember that over-the-counter (OTC) treatments can affect physical awareness and the ability to react and respond to emergencies. The following are some examples of physical disruptions that could affect your performance:

- A leg sprain or strain may cause difficulty in moving your foot from the accelerator to the brake, thus delaying reaction time.
- Gastrointestinal distress may cause you to become less focused and attentive to detail or to rush your actions.
- A cold or flu may be associated with distracting symptoms such as a runny nose, which can lead to loss of focus; the use of OTC medications can impair your ability to operate the vehicle safely.
- Headaches, especially migraine headaches, may cause changes in vision and hearing, which can severely diminish your ability to operate an emergency vehicle.

Attitude

A person's attitude is a key component of mental preparedness for emergency vehicle operation. Many people feel empowered and confident when they use lights and sirens as the driver of an emergency vehicle. These feelings of empowerment and confidence may lead to angry and aggressive driving, which can lead vehicle operators to take chances that they would not otherwise take, jeopardizing providers and patients. Aggressive driving can lead to serious injury or even death. There is no excuse for aggressive driving, even when other drivers are not reacting to your approach as legally required. As a professional, it is your job to focus on your driving, be cautious, and refuse to allow emotions to guide you behind the wheel.

A related issue concerns those vehicle operators who feel that because they already know how to drive, there is nothing to teach them that they do not already know. This type of attitude is misguided, as it is critical that vehicle operators know and understand the unique hazards inherent in operating an emergency vehicle. Avoiding aggressive driving and having a safety-first attitude are central to safe vehicle operation.

Safety Equipment

Emergency vehicles are equipped with safety equipment, such as seatbelts and airbags. Proper use of this equipment is essential to ensure the safety of vehicle operators, technicians, EMS providers, and the patients they transport.

Seatbelts

Seatbelts are an extremely effective method of reducing injuries and deaths from vehicle collisions. Over 15,000 lives are saved each year by proper use of seatbelts, and most EMS organizations have polices requiring the use of seatbelts in emergency vehicles.

For seatbelts to be effective, they must be worn properly. The lap belt needs to be placed snugly over the hips. The shoulder belt should be placed over the shoulder and diagonally across the torso away from the neck **FIGURE 2-3**. The shoulder belt should never be placed under the arm. Shorter or taller individuals may need to adjust the seatbelt restraint system or the position of the seat to ensure that the seatbelt fits properly. In older vehicles with separate lap and shoulder restraints, both systems must be used. Wearing a safety belt improperly may increase the risk of injury to a level similar to that of not wearing a seatbelt at all.

| Correct | Incorrect |

Figure 2-3 Proper seatbelt use.
© Jones & Bartlett Learning.

Although the evidence is overwhelming that seatbelts save lives, many people still do not wear them, including people working in EMS. Providers may think it is acceptable to stand or move around unrestrained in the patient compartment when the vehicle is in motion. Even those who have witnessed the often tragic consequences of not wearing a seatbelt may rationalize this practice, but unrestrained providers providing patient care are at significant risk for injury and death in the event of a collision.

As the emergency vehicle operator, you are responsible for ensuring that everyone is wearing a seatbelt properly before moving the vehicle. This includes providers in the patient compartment. Unrestrained or improperly restrained EMS providers die or are seriously injured each year in motor vehicle collisions. Even though it is legal, it is not safe practice for EMS providers to be unrestrained, even when providing patient care.

SAFETY POINTER

The single most important factor in seatbelt use is personal commitment. Make a commitment to ensure your safety first.

It may be more difficult or inconvenient to provide patient care while wearing a seatbelt, but this is no excuse to not wear one. Research is under way to develop a more ergonomic work space that will allow providers to tend to patients while being restrained. Regardless of the system in place, the vehicle operator must be properly restrained and ensure that all crew members are wearing seatbelts. This simple step can mean the difference between a minor injury and death in the event of a motor vehicle collision. Recommendations for developing a policy for seatbelt use in the ambulance are included in Chapter 12.

SAFETY POINTER

Seatbelts save lives. There is no excuse for not using seatbelts in the front compartment. Moreover, they should be used in the patient compartment.

Airbags

Airbags are important safety features that help to reduce **morbidity** and **mortality** in the event of a collision. Frontal airbags in emergency vehicles are usually located in the steering wheel or the dash and are designed to protect the occupant from hitting the steering wheel, dash, and windshield. Newer ambulances may include other types of airbags such as side curtain airbags, rollover airbags, knee bolsters, carpet airbags, and/or anti-slide airbags.

Vehicle occupants should be a safe distance from the airbag (at least 10 inches). No objects, including mobile data terminals or other devices, should obstruct the path between the occupant and the airbag. Objects located in this path during airbag deployment could interfere with the release of the airbag or become projectiles and cause further injury. It is important to remember that airbags are only part of the occupant safety system and that proper seatbelt use is required.

Headrests or Head Restraints

Head restraints, more commonly called headrests, in emergency vehicles vary depending on the make, model, and year of the vehicle. When available, they may help to reduce neck injuries in the event of a rear-end collision. Many drivers have improperly adjusted head restraints. The most common error is head restraints that are adjusted too low. A head restraint should be positioned no more than 2 inches behind the driver's head, with the center of the headrest at approximately ear level. When adjusted properly, the driver's head should contact the head restraint before the neck does. Properly positioning the head restraint may reduce whiplash and other neck injuries in the event of a rear-end collision.

Mirrors

Properly adjusted mirrors are important to safe vehicle operation. It is the emergency vehicle operator's responsibility to ensure the mirrors are positioned to maximize the operator's field of vision and limit blind spots. Mirrors may need to be adjusted multiple times during a shift in situations where drivers change frequently.

It is important to remember that even when you have properly maximized your field of vision, blind spots are still present behind the vehicle. To back the vehicle safely, use a spotter to provide directions. Services should have strict policies requiring use of a spotter when backing a vehicle. Recommended backing protocols can be found in Chapter 12.

SAFETY POINTER

Being safe is a personal commitment and is a *must* for every emergency vehicle operator. Be committed to your safety and the safety of others.

Helmets

When an ambulance is involved in a collision or evasive maneuver, unrestrained providers may fall and strike their heads. Unrestrained equipment such as oxygen gauges or suction unit bottles may become airborne and strike providers, and sharp corners or edges may cause injuries. Thus, some safety experts advocate the use of safety helmets for EMS personnel during patient transport.

Dr. Nadine Levick, CEO of Objective Safety and Research Director of EMS Safety Foundation, reports that 74% of EMS fatalities are the result of vehicle collisions and that 64% of those deaths are the result of serious head injuries. It is logical to presume that helmets could help reduce morbidity and mortality in these situations. Specially designed helmets for protecting EMS personnel have yet to be developed, and traditional fire helmets would not be effective for this purpose. The use of helmets, however, would not reduce the need to improve ambulance design and testing for greater safety. Routine helmet use will require further education, training, positive reinforcement, and practical policies implemented by visionary leaders who are committed to safety and research.

Equipment Security

Properly securing equipment is essential to prevent it from becoming a projectile during a collision or sudden stop. Unsecured equipment such as first-in bags (jump kits), oxygen caddies, defibrillators, or monitors may become deadly projectiles and have been documented to cause provider and patient injury. Equipment should always be secured in cabinets or in specifically designed locations. One method of securing gear is to attach carabineers to the bag and clip it to a specified location in the box. Properly securing equipment takes only a few seconds; there is simply no justifiable reason to leave equipment unsecured. Ambulances should be properly equipped with monitor locks and computer docking stations to secure equipment in a usable position.

SAFETY POINTER

Gear should always be secured in a compartment or specified location.

Patient Safety

When patients call an ambulance, they expect to be transported safely. Remember rule number one: Do no harm. You should never put a patient in jeopardy during transport. One essential way to ensure patient safety is through proper use of stretcher restraints.

Many providers assume that when a patient is secured on the stretcher with three lap belts and the stretcher is properly latched to the floor, the patient is safe. Unfortunately, this is not true. Patients should always be secured to the stretcher using a four-point shoulder harness with a chest strap, a pelvis strap, and a leg strap FIGURE 2-4 .

Stretcher manufacturers now generally include a four-point shoulder harness as part of their standard equipment. Many

Figure 2-4 Proper patient restraints.
© Jones & Bartlett Learning.

providers believe that the shoulder harnesses are optional, but in fact, they are critical for ensuring that the patient does not slide out of the stretcher straps during a collision. It is imperative that providers use the manufacturer's specifications for securing patients; failure to do so could result in increased liability for injuries in the case of a collision. The scenario at the beginning of this chapter is a good example of this happening. When the shoulder harnesses are properly secured in accordance with the manufacturer's recommendations, they should not interfere with your ability to provide patient care, including a 12-lead ECG or other monitoring.

SAFETY POINTER

You have the responsibility to ensure that your patients are properly secured. In many instances, patients who were improperly secured without the use of the provided shoulder harnesses have been killed or severely injured following a vehicle collision. Your patient's safety is your responsibility.

The stretcher should be secured to the floor during transport. Slightly raise the head end to help prevent the patient from hitting the captain's seat or bulkhead in the event of a frontal impact crash. Note, however, that even when properly secured, ambulance crash tests have revealed that stretchers can detach from the mounts and become projectiles in the event of a collision. It is interesting to note that in the United States, the locking system of the most commonly used stretchers and mounting systems is designed to withstand only 2,200 foot-pounds of force—roughly equivalent to only 74 pounds moving at 30 mph. In addition, stretchers are secured at only a single point of contact on a rack that prevents the wheels from rolling too far forward. This design is significantly inferior to stretchers used in

Europe. In Europe, stretchers and their mounting systems are able to endure loads 10 times the force of gravity over a crash impulse window of less than 100 milliseconds without failure. Further, stretchers are secured to the floor at three points of contact, each of which restrains motion on at least two axes.

Passenger Safety

Family members and friends often want to accompany patients in the ambulance. Your company should have a policy for this case, and you should be familiar with the policy to ensure that this is an approved practice.

An adult passenger should be transported in the front passenger seat and wear a seatbelt. The emergency vehicle operator should assist the passenger into the front seat and ensure that the seatbelt is properly attached. The emergency vehicle operator should also assist the passenger out of the vehicle upon arrival at the destination. Any passenger who refuses to wear a seatbelt should not be permitted to ride in the ambulance. Small folding stools may be useful to help passengers into and out of the passenger seat. These stools may be stored behind the passenger seat of the ambulance.

EMS providers should not allow themselves to become distracted by conversing with accompanying family members or friends. The primary objective is getting to the hospital safely, and this may require the operator's full attention. It is not discourteous to inform passengers that you are unable to talk while driving to ensure that everyone arrives safely at their destination.

While in general, passengers should be seated in the front compartment, there are certain circumstances in which it may be advantageous for a passenger to ride in the patient compartment. For example, it may be beneficial for a parent to ride in the patient compartment to provide support to a pediatric patient. In this event, the child must be properly restrained in accordance with his or her age and size and with local laws. Children should never be transported on the parent's lap, even if the parent is secured to the stretcher. Parents in the patient compartment must also be properly restrained.

Prior to allowing the parent to ride with the patient, a member of the crew should explain any necessary interventions so that the parent knows what to expect during transport. Parents who are overly emotional or unable to control themselves should not be permitted to ride in the patient compartment. Family members or friends should never be transported in the patient

SAFETY POINTER

EMS providers should never sit on the end of the stretcher to provide patient care during transport. This practice places the patient at risk of being injured by the provider should a vehicle collision occur.

compartment when the patient is in respiratory or cardiac arrest or when other critical conditions exist.

In special situations, children may need to be transported as passengers when their parent is a patient. This practice should be limited to situations in which no other options exist. Children who are eligible to ride in the passenger seat according to your state law should ride in the passenger seat with proper restraints. Children who require a safety seat must be transported in a child safety seat or booster seat. Safety seats may not be placed on side-facing seats. Children who are not required to use a child safety seat of any kind may ride in the captain's seat (rear-facing seat) with a seatbelt, based on your department's policy.

When necessary, additional emergency responders may be transported as passengers. It is the responsibility of the emergency vehicle operator to ensure that they are properly restrained the same as any other crew member. Remember that the number of occupants should never exceed the number of seatbelts in the vehicle.

Roadside Safety

Many emergency incidents occur on interstates, highways, and other roadways. An emergency scene on the roadway presents unique hazards to the emergency vehicle operator. Every year, many EMS providers are injured or killed at roadway incidents.

Motorists may be distracted by the scene and not paying attention to their driving. When drivers see the lights on an accident scene, they are likely to drive toward it because our hands follow our eyes. The safest place for an emergency vehicle responding to a highway incident is off of the roadway and away from traffic. Emergency vehicle operators need to ensure they are seen by other motorists and have been given the right of way. Whenever possible, you should avoid working on a roadway or highway or at least aim to limit the amount of time you spend on the roadway as much as possible, even if it means delaying patient care until you can move to a safe location. When it is necessary to work on a roadway, you should take proper precautions:

- Establish a safe work zone by having the police or fire department block traffic and using traffic-control devices FIGURE 2-5.
- Position the vehicle properly ("downstream" of the collision).
- Consider the use of warning lights.
- Wear high-visibility apparel.

Safe Work Zone

Emergency vehicles can be positioned to establish a safe work zone by blocking traffic and providing protection for personnel operating at the emergency scene. Ideally, fire apparatus should be used to block traffic. Cones and traffic warning devices should be used to warn unsuspecting motorists at extended incidents whenever possible. The key is having the first-arriving unit block traffic from the scene. It is not ideal for the ambulance to perform

Figure 2-5 Proper traffic blocking techniques and high-visibility gear will help to keep you safe.
© Mike Legeros. Used with permission.

this function, but it is needed to secure the scene and warn oncoming drivers. The preferred placement of the ambulance is in front (downstream) of the collision, which limits exposure to moving traffic during patient loading. It is also the best position for egress once it is time to transport the patient.

If an ambulance is being used to block traffic, angle the vehicle so that it is aimed away from the scene, with the rear doors not directly facing on-coming traffic. Keep the rear doors closed so that the vehicle's lights are visible. This positioning provides additional protection so that providers can access equipment. In addition, turn the vehicle's wheels away from the work zone so that in the event it is struck by a motorist from behind, it will not directly collide with the scene. Note that the patient should not be loaded into the vehicle until it is moved around the incident and positioned such that the collision scene serves as a protective barrier.

At high-risk incidents and incident locations, it may be necessary to request assistance from additional responders (e.g., police, fire, EMS, and highway services) to ensure scene safety. The Traffic Incident Management (TIM) system can help responders coordinate their efforts when more than one response vehicle is necessary at an incident to avoid placing the ambulance in an area that may be blocked by other emergency vehicles.

The TIM system comprises several components that both allow traffic to move safely and smoothly around an emergency scene and allow the first responders to work in a relatively safe environment FIGURE 2-6. The system is made up of the following:

- *Advanced warning area.* This area gives motorists ample warning of an incident ahead and is usually marked with a *pink* diamond-shaped warning sign placed by the first unit arriving on scene.
- *Transition area.* This area begins the flare or cone pattern, which is used to taper the number of lanes and move traffic away from the incident.
- *Buffer space.* This area starts to slow traffic and funnel it away from the incident.

Figure 2-6 The traffic incident management system.
Courtesy of FAAC, Inc. Based on original figure by Emergency Responder Safety Institute.

- *Protection vehicles.* This area is directly "upstream" from the incident. Vehicles positioned here are primarily used for blocking and secondarily used as resource vehicles. "Lane + 1 blocking" affords a good work space for rescuers and a "shadow" area that limits drivers' ability to rubberneck. Position vehicles to both block and direct traffic.
- *Work space.* This is the area of the incident, and it must remain as open and as safe as possible. Protection vehicles may have to be repositioned as the operation progresses to maintain a high level of safety while allowing traffic to flow with as little impediment as possible.
- *Termination area.* This is the area immediately downstream of the incident that allows traffic to continue to move in a controlled manner. This area should be avoided by rescuers at all times and at all costs. If the incident dictates that rescuers enter into the termination area, then the work space should be extended and the termination area moved further downstream. This area can be used for staging of tow trucks, medical examiner vehicles, and other ancillary vehicles that are not actively engaged in the rescue process.

SAFETY POINTER

Become familiar with the Traffic Incident Management (TIM) system. If you have any questions about vehicle placement, consult with the incident commander who has overall responsibility for scene safety and comprehensive knowledge about the operations.

For more in-depth information regarding the TIM system, visit the Emergency Responder Safety Institute website.

Vehicle Positioning

It is important to position the emergency vehicle properly at an emergency scene to ensure the safety of motorists, patients, and providers. Consider the location of the incident and unique hazards, such as inclement weather and poor visibility, when determining the safest places to position the vehicle. For example, vehicles should not be placed on corners, at the crest of hills, or in blind spots. Providers need to be aware of the unique hazards within their response district.

When staging the vehicle at a scene, several issues may need to be taken into account in the placement of the vehicle, not only for safe scene operations but also for easy egress once scene management is complete. Examples include placing vehicles uphill from spilled liquids and vapors, downwind from fumes and smoke, upstream when first on scene, and downstream when on scene with other units and loading patients. Vigilance should be used when positioning the ambulance so as not to get blocked in by additional emergency vehicles, prohibiting rapid transport from the scene.

A majority of emergency responses occur at a residence or other locations where there is a driveway. In these instances, the driveway is usually the safest place to park the ambulance. When arriving at the incident location, depending on the situation and priority of the assignment, your partner should exit the vehicle wearing high-visibility apparel and serve as a spotter to help you back into the driveway. In some situations, it may be necessary to park at the curb in front of the residence. Either way, once the vehicle is parked, the emergency lights

OPERATOR INCIDENT

In southwestern Colorado in March 2007, several teenagers were killed due to improper parking and misuse of warning equipment by an emergency provider at the scene. A deputy investigating a car off the road drove past a collision on a curve and parked without using emergency lights, leaving his headlights on. The deputy parked to the right of the travel lanes and left of the disabled vehicle. This created an optical illusion with the stopped car, creating the appearance that the oncoming lane was further right than it really was. As a result, the fatigued driver of an oncoming utility truck drove into the scene on the shoulder, striking the teenagers inside of and around the disabled vehicle. The truck driver saw the deputy's headlights and mistakenly thought the deputy was in the approaching lane. Had the deputy used his emergency lights, turned off the headlights, or lit the scene properly, this incident may have been avoided.

and headlights should be turned off if they might interfere with the normal flow of traffic in any way.

Warning Lights

It may seem counterintuitive, but emergency lights may actually be a safety hazard. It is not uncommon for motorists to crash into parked emergency vehicles that have warning lights operating. The flashing lights attract the drivers' attention, which may lead them to steer toward the emergency vehicle. When possible, warning lights should be limited to amber lights in an alternating pattern on the vehicle's corners. When this lighting option is not available, the vehicle's hazard lights should be used. Drivers are accustomed to seeing yellow or hazard lights and recognize that they need to slow down and proceed with caution. Most drivers are not accustomed to emergency lighting and may be distracted by the lights and unsure how to respond. Today, most states require blue lights on the rear portion of all emergency vehicles. Provided your specific state does not prohibit the use of a blue light, this is a helpful recommendation.

The use of warning lights for blocking vehicles is discussed in detail in NFPA 1451, *Standard for a Fire and Emergency Service Vehicle Operations Training Program*.

High-Visibility Apparel

High-visibility apparel increases the provider's visibility when working along a roadway. Federal law requires all workers within the right of way along a federal highway to wear an ANSI 107 (2004) Class 2 or 3 high-visibility vest. This law applies to all first responders, though exceptions do exist for police personnel based on tactical need. The use of high-visibility vests increases personnel visibility and reduces the risk of severe injury or death **FIGURE 2-7**. These vests are also required to come with a five-point breakaway feature for safety. However, it is important to understand that the use of high-visibility apparel alone does not make you safe.

Figure 2-7   Agencies should obtain high-visibility vests (ANSI-107 [2004] Class 2 or 3 garments or ANSI-207 [2006]-compliant garments) for their personnel. Ensure that vests are sized to fit when worn on top of full turnout gear, such as in cold-weather situations, responses to motor vehicle crashes where there is no fire, or where otherwise appropriate.
© Nancy G Fire Photography, Nancy Greifenhagen/Alamy.

SAFETY POINTER

Place approved high-visibility apparel in an easily accessible location. Use positive reinforcement and lead by example so that wearing high-visibility apparel becomes the norm.

Mechanical Problems

As an emergency vehicle operator, you may encounter situations that involve safety hazards such as a mechanical problem or vehicle fire. In these situations, the overriding concern should be your personal safety and the safety of your partner, patient, and passengers.

Common mechanical problems such as engine failure, transmission failure, an overheating vehicle, or a flat tire can create an unexpected and hazardous situation. When a mechanical problem occurs, every attempt should be made to move the vehicle away from traffic. If your vehicle is blocking traffic in any way, immediately turn on your hazard lights to warn oncoming motorists. Do not use your emergency lights, as this may confuse drivers who associate the emergency lights with an incident such as a motor vehicle collision. After turning on your hazard lights, you should request assistance to control the traffic hazard in accordance with your agency's policies. Remember to request an additional unit to transport your patient, if necessary.

SAFETY POINTER

Take precautions to protect yourself in the event of mechanical difficulties:
- Move the vehicle away from traffic.
- Put on the vehicle's hazard lights.
- Call for assistance.
- Safely exit the vehicle.
- Use traffic-control devices.

Once assistance has been requested, you should don high-visibility apparel and exit the vehicle. To provide additional protection and warn oncoming traffic, you should set up flares, warning triangles, or other traffic-control devices. Whenever possible, place warning devices at least 300 feet from the vehicle in equal increments to direct traffic away from the disabled vehicle. Roadside repairs should never be attempted by nonqualified personnel; always defer to local policies. Keep in mind that flares may create additional danger if there are leaking fluids on the ground.

Although rare, vehicle fires can occur in an emergency medical vehicle. Emergency medical units carry oxygen, which is an accelerant and can be extremely dangerous in the event of a fire. If a vehicle fire occurs, you must rapidly assess the situation and take actions to maximize safety. The priority should be removing the patient from the vehicle. If the vehicle is on fire, you should not take time to remove equipment. Since the oxygen system on board could result in an explosion, your main concern is to move yourself and the patient a safe distance away from the vehicle.

SAFETY POINTER

Safety is the number one priority during an unexpected or hazardous situation.

WRAP-UP

Summary

- The priority for EMS providers is to ensure their own safety and the safety of their partner, patients, and passengers.
- Having a safety-first attitude is a critical component of safe vehicle operation.
- Safety is a habit and a culture that relies on personal responsibility and commitment to excellence.
- Mental and physical preparedness includes efforts to reduce or avoid sleep deprivation, stress, extreme emotions, or physical ailments, which may inhibit decision making.
- To be effective, a seatbelt must be placed properly, with the lap belt snug over the hips and the shoulder belt over the shoulder and diagonally across the torso.
- Care providers must always be properly restrained during transport, even when they are providing care to the patient in the patient compartment.
- Emergency vehicle airbags located in the steering wheel or dash are designed to protect the driver and front passenger in the event of a collision.

- Properly positioned headrests can reduce the risk of neck injuries.
- Correct mirror positioning and use of spotters when backing are important safety precautions.
- It is necessary to secure all equipment to avoid projectiles if the vehicle stops suddenly.
- Patients should always be secured to the stretcher using a four-point shoulder harness with chest strap, pelvis strap, and leg strap.
- Adult passengers should ride in the front passenger seat with a seatbelt.
- Children should always be properly restrained according to their age, size, and weight in accordance with state guidelines.
- To establish a safe work zone in the event of a roadway incident, position the vehicle properly, consider the use of warning lights, and wear high-visibility apparel.
- In the event of a mechanical failure, move the vehicle away from traffic, use hazard lights, call for assistance, safely exit the vehicle, and use traffic-control devices.

Glossary

morbidity   Illness or harm; a diseased state.

mortality   Death; the quality of being mortal.

sleep deprivation   The state of having insufficient sleep.

Additional Resources

Emergency Responder Safety Institute, http://www.respondersafety.com
National Highway Traffic Safety Administration, http://www.nhtsa.gov
National Safety Council, http://www.nsc.org

U.S. Department of Labor: Occupational Safety and Health Administration (OSHA), http://www.osha.gov

References

1. McCallion, T. (2012). Consider the dangers of shift work: It's important to have a fatigue management plan in place. *Journal of Emergency Medical Services*. Retrieved from http://www.jems.com/article/emsinsider/consider-dangers-shift-work

2. National Fire Protection Association. (2013). *NFPA 1451: Standard for a fire and emergency services vehicle operations training program*. Quincy, MA: Author, 2013.

3. National Sleep Foundation. (2005). *2005 sleep in America poll: Summary of findings.* Retrieved from https://sleepfoundation .org/sites/default/files/2005_summary_of_findings.pdf

4. National Sleep Foundation. (2009). *2009 sleep in America poll: Summary of findings.* Retrieved from https://sleepfoundation .org/sites/default/files/2009%20SLEEP%20IN%20AMERICA%20 SOF%20EMBARGOED_0.PDF

5. National Sleep Foundation. (2015). *Facts and stats: Drowsy driving – Stay alert, arrive alive.* Retrieved from http://drowsydriving.org /about/facts-and-stats/

6. Proudfoot, S. L. (2005). Ambulance crashes: Fatality factors for EMS workers. *EMS World.* Retrieved from http://www .emsworld.com/article/10323905/ambulance-crashes-fatality -factors-for-ems-workers

7. U.S. Department of Homeland Security Science and Technology Directorate, First Responders Group. (2015). *Ambulance patient compartment human factors design guidebook.* Retrieved from http://www.firstresponder.gov/TechnologyDocuments /Ambulance%20Patient%20Compartment%20Human%20 Factors%20Design%20Guidebook.pdf

CHAPTER 3

EMS Vehicle Operation and the Law

OBJECTIVES

3.1 Define the types of laws that affect EMS vehicle operation.

3.2 Explain the legal terms related to EMS vehicle operation.

3.3 Describe the appropriate use of lights and sirens.

3.4 Discuss safety considerations for responding to an emergency scene.

3.5 Outline the types of preventable collisions most common to emergency vehicle operations.

3.6 Discuss the assessment of liability and how liability affects the emergency vehicle operator.

3.7 Explain steps the emergency vehicle operator can take to avoid legal entanglements.

3.8 Describe how to respond appropriately in the event of a collision.

SCENARIO

You and your partner are at the daily meeting in the center of town when a Priority 1 response is dispatched for your zone. As you drive past the airport, with your lights and siren on, you approach a red traffic light. There is no traffic to the left and a few vehicles to your right. Though they have a green light, they are stopped at the intersection. You slow down slightly and proceed through the intersection. Suddenly, almost out of nowhere, a BMW pulls directly in front of your ambulance from the right. You react quickly and hit the brakes, but your vehicle hits the driver's side door.

You are unharmed. You quickly check on your partner; he says he is okay but that his sternum is sore. Next, you get out to check on the driver of the other vehicle. She is conscious, alert, and oriented. Her left leg appears to be broken. She also appears to be trapped in the vehicle and will require extrication.

You notify dispatch to assign another ambulance to the original call and request that police, fire rescue, an ambulance, and a supervisor come to your crash scene. An additional ambulance arrives to take both you and your partner to the hospital, but you are both discharged after a few hours with only minor bruising. The front end of the ambulance has significant damage and will be out of service until it can be repaired. Local media picks up the story and your name appears in the newspaper. You are interviewed by the town's police traffic safety unit, which will be investigating the incident. According to your service's policy, all crashes are investigated by police traffic safety, and they ultimately issue a report if there was fault or a need for education or retraining. Witnesses report that the driver of the BMW was talking on her cell phone prior to the collision. The police department will not be issuing a report, but the town attorney's office is notified that the driver has brought a $7 million lawsuit against your service. You must hire an attorney because you are personally named in the suit. Eventually, all parties agree to a settlement after a long and difficult legal battle.

1. How often do you review and have trainings on local driving laws?
2. What are your standard operating procedures, protocols, and/or responsibilities when you witness or are involved in a collision?

Introduction

This chapter introduces the legal considerations for emergency vehicle operators. Service policy makers and their driver trainers should outline very clearly what your responsibilities are for operating the emergency vehicle. They should also provide high-quality training to you to prepare you for your job. Department leadership should also remain current with all laws and policies that pertain to driving emergency vehicles in your jurisdiction. However, it is ultimately your responsibility to properly perform your job and know the laws that govern your actions. If you are involved in a crash in which someone is seriously injured or killed and you broke traffic laws, violated department standard operating procedures (SOPs), or acted without due regard to others (a subject discussed later), you could face legal consequences, possibly even manslaughter or negligent homicide charges in the case of a fatality.

SAFETY POINTER

The vehicle operator should be familiar with the state traffic laws, specific municipality ordinances, and all department rules related to emergency vehicle operation.

Criminal and Civil Law

The U.S. judicial system is divided into two primary types of law, criminal and civil.

Criminal law involves determining whether a statute has been violated and, if so, assessing an appropriate punishment, whether that be a fine, jail or prison incarceration, or both. For a minor criminal offense, such as illegally parking your ambulance when not on an emergency call, a police officer could issue a citation requiring you to appear in front of a judge, who would most likely impose a fine. For a more serious criminal offense, such as striking and killing a pedestrian, the vehicle operator could be arrested and placed in jail and would need to arrange for legal representation in the ensuing criminal proceedings.

Motor vehicle laws involve the criminal justice system. If you violate a traffic law, such as exceeding the speed limit in your personal vehicle, you have committed a criminal offense. While emergency vehicles are given a certain amount of latitude with regard to following all motor vehicle laws, emergency vehicle operators may still be ticketed or fined if they disregard these laws and put the public at risk.

Civil law is much broader and more often invoked against a vehicle operator in cases of vehicle collisions (even when the incident does not lead to criminal charges). In a civil action, an injured person files a lawsuit naming the vehicle operator as the **defendant**. The **plaintiff** (person suing) asks for monetary compensation for his or her physical, emotional, and psychological injuries as well as other damages, such as loss of employability or other financial harm.

In criminal cases, the state (or prosecution) must prove to a jury that the accused is guilty of the crime beyond a **reasonable doubt**, meaning that a reasonable person would not doubt the accused party's guilt. In civil cases, however, the plaintiff must prove his or her case based on only a **preponderance of the evidence**, meaning there is slightly more evidence of guilt than of innocence. In a civil case, the jury may choose to award the plaintiff compensation from the defendant at the requested amount or at a higher or lower amount, based on the jury's determination of the defendant's level of guilt.

Legal Terms

The most common cause of legal trouble for a vehicle operator is a collision. In a vehicle collision there may be criminal charges brought against the operator, but much more likely there will be a civil suit naming the operator as a defendant. In civil suits involving collisions, the primary goal is to establish **liability**, which is the determination of who is primarily at fault for the collision. In civil cases involving emergency vehicles, the primary determination of liability is based on a term called **negligence**, which indicates that the vehicle operator did not perform his or her responsibilities correctly. To prove negligence in a vehicle collision, the plaintiff must prove that the defendant had a responsibility to act in a certain way and that he or she failed to do so, resulting in a collision that caused injury to the plaintiff.

Gross negligence is a more serious form of negligence, and implies reckless conduct and a blatant disregard for the safety and lives of others. Consider, for example, a vehicle operator driving under the influence of alcohol who collides with a vehicle that is stopped at an intersection and kills the vehicle's driver upon impact. To prove gross negligence, the plaintiff would need to prove that the defendant's conduct was deliberately reckless and without concern for other drivers' safety. The line between negligence and gross negligence can be unclear and may need to be determined by a court.

In the event of a collision involving an EMS vehicle, a court primarily bases its judgment on these two questions:

1. Did the emergency vehicle operator have reasonable grounds to believe he or she was responding to a *true emergency*?
2. Did the emergency vehicle operator exercise *due regard* for the safety of others?

A **true emergency** is a situation in which there is a high probability of death or serious injury to an individual or of significant property loss, and the actions of the responders can mitigate the situation. **Due regard** refers to taking appropriate considerations in a given situation. The determination of "appropriate" is based on what a reasonably careful person could be expected to do if he or she were performing similar duties under similar circumstances. Thus, "due regard for the safety of others" means taking precautions that a reasonably prudent person would take to safeguard the public in a similar situation.

OPERATOR INCIDENT

The following comparisons are loosely based on incidents that tragically occur somewhere almost every day. Note how differently the incident appears to the public when it involves an ambulance.

In a small suburban neighborhood, there was a tragic crash that involved a preschool-aged child on a big wheel, who rolled down his driveway and entered the street. A pine tree at the foot of the driveway was a potential obstruction to the view of the oncoming traffic. Two middle-aged couples were in a car traveling through this suburban neighborhood on their way to dinner. They were traveling at the posted speed limit. The child suddenly darted out in front of them, and they did not see the child before striking and fatally injuring him. While EMS was attempting to resuscitate the child, police took statements from witnesses, did a field sobriety test, and checked for skid marks as a part of their investigation. In the end, there was no ticket issued because it was determined that the vehicle could not have avoided hitting the child.

In another collision a few months later in a different small community, an ambulance was responding to a call on a residential street. They were exceeding the posted speed limit but not by more than the 10 mph that their company policy allows. A school-aged child rode his bicycle into the side of the ambulance. He was not wearing a helmet and he too was fatally injured. The EMS crew tried to revive the child, but they were unsuccessful. The police again interviewed witnesses, measured skid marks, and did a field sobriety test. In this case, although no evidence appeared to indicate that the EMS crew was at fault and no tickets were issued, the case was turned over to the grand jury for further investigation. The media attacked the EMS service and published the name and address of the emergency vehicle operator. In the end, the grand jury determined that the crash could not have been avoided and the emergency vehicle operator was not at fault, but the service's and operator's reputations were deeply damaged.

As you can see from these two similar cases, the due regard provision sets a higher standard for EMS providers. Always make every effort to take due regard for the safety of others while operating an EMS vehicle.

The law gives a tremendous amount of responsibility to emergency vehicle operators when a call is classified as a true emergency; however, operators must still show due regard for the safety of all others. To show due regard, the emergency vehicle operator must give sufficient notice of the vehicle's approach (e.g., lights and sirens) to allow other motorists and pedestrians to clear a path and protect themselves. If you do not give notice of your approach until a collision is unavoidable, you have not satisfied the principle of due regard for the safety of others.

Figure 3-1 Emergency warning devices should be used when taking any exemptions to vehicle and traffic laws.
© Karin Hildebrand Lau/Alamy.

SAFETY POINTER

The emergency vehicle operator is held to a higher standard than all other drivers on the road.

Use of Lights and Siren

Lights and sirens are used to alert motorists and pedestrians of the approach of an emergency vehicle. State laws mandate that the emergency vehicle operator use emergency warning devices such as lights and/or siren, when reasonably necessary, especially when taking advantage of any traffic law exemptions FIGURE 3-1 . However, the use of signaling equipment does not guarantee that motorists and pedestrians are aware of the presence of the vehicle, nor do they protect the vehicle operator from civil or criminal liability if a collision occurs.

SAFETY POINTER

Legally your emergency warning devices require traffic to yield the right of way. However, you have no guarantee that you will receive it. Motorists or pedestrians who do not give you the right of way are breaking the law, but you are still required to give them due regard!

The use of emergency lights must comply with state and local laws, state and local EMS rules and regulations, and your company's policy. The lights do not provide as much protection or warning as you may think. Furthermore, in parking at the scene of an emergency, the use of the warning lights may actually make the scene unsafe and draw other motorists' vehicles toward your location. It is important to remember that low sun, glare, fog, and tinted windows in other vehicles can reduce the effectiveness of warning lights.

At night, red warning lights may blend in with other red lights in traffic or the neon light along the side of the streets. Warning lights mounted on top of a vehicle may not be visible in the rearview mirror of vehicles in front of the emergency vehicle.

There are similar concerns with the effectiveness of the siren. In general, sirens can be heard only to a distance of 230 feet ahead of the vehicle. At speeds greater than 40 mph, you can completely outrun the effectiveness of your siren. Even at close range, the siren may not be heard by a motorist who has the vehicle's windows closed and is using the air conditioning or radio. Newer cars even advertise how much outside noise the car blocks, and this includes emergency vehicle's sirens.

SAFETY POINTER

Do not overestimate the reach of your emergency warning devices.

Responding Safely

When responding to an incident, emergency vehicle operators should be made aware if they are being dispatched on a potential emergency. Dispatch should obtain information from the caller to determine how the vehicle operator should respond (i.e., emergency or non-emergency) by using an emergency medical dispatch system. EMS system directors may be liable if they do not have a policy regarding what information responders should receive when they are dispatched.

Nonemergency responses include incidents involving chronic illness (without life-threatening complications), minor injuries, and stable patients. True emergencies include cardiac or respiratory complications, major trauma, or other complaints based on your system's 9-1-1 dispatch categories. In EMS systems, the emergency vehicle operator should initiate a high-priority response to a presumed, true emergency that includes the use of emergency warning devices. The response mode may change or downgrade if a first responder reports that the call does not involve a life-threatening situation.

The decision about routine or emergency transport should be made by asking the following questions:

- Will the time saved make a significant difference in the patient's outcome?
- Will emergency transport create an unnecessarily unsafe situation for the public, myself and my partner(s), and the patient?
- What effect will the emergency warning devices have on the surrounding public, patient, driver, and crew?

It is important to note that in situations in which it is necessary to respond to the station or emergency scene in your own private vehicle, you must adhere to all applicable motor vehicle laws. Privately owned nonemergency vehicles are not granted any exemptions or special privileges by most states and must obey all state vehicle and traffic laws, even when states allow the use of emergency warning devices. State rules and department policies vary greatly in what they consider an authorized emergency vehicle. Regardless, if you are responding in a nonemergency vehicle, you should be careful not to let the excitement affect your driving and should make a special effort to drive in a safe manner. As with emergency vehicles, you should pay close attention to speed limits, road and weather conditions, intersections, and maneuvering your vehicle around the emergency scene.

If your private vehicle has an emergency identification light, you must comply with the applicable emergency motor vehicle rules and regulations that cover size, type, color, and candle power of the light. You must also recognize that you are representing your emergency response organization and drawing attention to yourself when you respond with a light on your private vehicle. You might consider shutting off the light when you are stopped at traffic lights or stop signs to avoid distracting motorists and pedestrians FIGURE 3-2 . Always follow the SOPs of your organization and any state laws concerning the use of colored lights on personal vehicles.

Figure 3-2 Private vehicles may be issued emergency warning devices for emergency response.
© Michael Matthews - Police Images/Alamy.

Types of Collisions

One of the most common causes of legal issues for an emergency vehicle operator is a collision involving the emergency vehicle he or she is driving. There are many types of collisions common to emergency vehicle operations. The ones most likely to involve legal trouble for the operator are preventable collisions.

A **preventable collision** is one in which the driver failed to do everything reasonable to prevent its occurrence. Note that the word *reasonable*, rather than *possible*, is used in this definition. There is always something possible that could have been done to prevent a collision (such as not responding to the call or taking another street). Reasonable preventive measures include knowing, understanding, and obeying traffic laws; adjusting speed to existing conditions; scanning ahead to anticipate stops; and anticipating the reactions of other drivers and pedestrians to your emergency vehicle.

There are many different types of preventable collisions:

- Parking collisions may result from double-parking, failure to warn traffic of your parked position, and parking in an unconventional location, to name a few examples.
- Intersection collisions are those that happen at stop lights, stop signs, or other intersections, where different directions of traffic must cross paths.
- Backing collisions occur while the vehicle is in reverse gear.
- In rear-end collisions, the emergency vehicle impacts a vehicle in front of it; these incidents are commonly caused by not maintaining a safe following distance, not looking ahead to anticipate the need to stop, or not controlling vehicle speed.
- Pedestrian collisions are always considered preventable, even though children and adults may perform sudden, unexpected maneuvers.
- Mechanical failure collisions are often the result of lack of attention during the vehicle inspection, reckless

SAFETY POINTER

You can be held both criminally and civilly liable if a collision occurs while you are on duty as an emergency responder. The agency for which you work can also be brought into a lawsuit if the case can be made that you were improperly or inadequately instructed or that no effort was made to control unsafe or reckless vehicle operation.

Figure 3-3 Collisions into stationary objects are considered preventable collisions.
© Jon Hill/The Lowell Sun/AP Photo.

or abusive vehicle handling, or operating the vehicle beyond its mechanical limits (e.g., over the gross vehicle weight rating).

- Adverse weather collisions may be caused by failure to drive according to the existing conditions, failure to postpone nonemergency calls, failure to use snow chains, or driving in adverse weather conditions.
- Traffic lane encroachment collisions may be the result of using improper passing techniques, weaving through or merging with traffic at unsafe times, or changing lanes in an unsafe manner.
- Collisions with fixed objects such as low overheads, buildings, poles, parked cars, and trees or collisions resulting from running off the roadway or overturning the vehicle may be caused by unsafe evasive action on the part of the emergency vehicle operator **FIGURE 3-3**.

Criminal and Civil Law
Liability in Cases of Collisions

As mentioned earlier, liability is the determination of who is primarily at fault in the event of a collision. In addition to evaluating whether the emergency vehicle was responding to a true emergency with due regard for the safety of others, the judge or jury may ask the following questions:

- Are there any state, national, or department standards for emergency vehicle operation that may apply? If so, did the specific emergency operator comply with them?
- Do any state statutes regarding emergency vehicle exemptions apply?
- Was the emergency vehicle operator properly trained and supervised per accepted standards, and did the operator follow the SOPs of the agency?
- Was the vehicle properly equipped, was the equipment being properly operated, and are there records of relevant repairs and preventive maintenance?

- Were the manufacturer's ratings exceeded?
- Did the emergency vehicle have seatbelts, and if so, were they properly utilized?

A finding of liability in a vehicle collision involving an ambulance will likely result in monetary damages being assessed to the vehicle operator, as well as the EMS service he or she represents. It is in everyone's best interest for the emergency vehicle operator to avoid any action that might result in a collision for which he or she might be liable.

Avoiding Legal Entanglements

Ultimately, it is your responsibility to know and obey the laws of your state and the SOPs of your organization as they relate to driving an emergency vehicle. State laws may vary regarding the maximum speed at which emergency vehicles can drive during an emergency operation and which traffic law exemptions emergency vehicles have, but in all states, emergency vehicle operators must drive with due regard for the safety of others. The best way to stay out of legal entanglements is to be attentive and practice safe driving.

If you do become involved in a collision, stay calm, follow your agency's SOP, and notify the police. Care for any injured persons immediately and always remain courteous and polite. You should not make any statements to the media but should cooperate with any investigations or police documentation **FIGURE 3-4**.

Figure 3-4 Always cooperate with a crash scene investigation.
© Valley News, photographer: Jennifer Hauck.

WRAP-UP

Summary

- Criminal law involves determining whether a statute has been violated and, if so, assessing an appropriate punishment, whether that be a fine, jail or prison incarceration, or both.
- Civil law is much broader and more often invoked against a vehicle operator in cases of vehicle collisions (even when the incident does not lead to criminal charges).
- In criminal cases, the state (or prosecution) must prove to a jury that the accused is guilty of the crime beyond a reasonable doubt, meaning that a reasonable person would not doubt the accused party's guilt.
- In civil cases, the plaintiff must prove his or her case based on only a preponderance of the evidence, meaning there is slightly more evidence of guilt than of innocence.
- A true emergency is a situation in which there is a high probability of death or serious injury to an individual or of significant property loss, and the actions of the responders can mitigate the situation.

- Due regard is taking appropriate considerations in a given situation. The determination of "appropriate" is based on what a reasonably careful person could be expected to do if he or she were performing similar duties under similar circumstances.
- Lights and sirens are used to alert motorists and pedestrians of the approach of an emergency vehicle. State laws mandate that the emergency vehicle operator use emergency warning devices such as lights and/or siren, when reasonably necessary, especially when taking advantage of any traffic law exemptions.
- A preventable collision is one in which the driver failed to do everything reasonable to prevent its occurrence. Note that the word *reasonable*, rather than *possible*, is used in this definition.
- The best way to stay out of legal entanglements is to be attentive and practice safe driving.

Glossary

civil law The type of law that pertains to determining responsibility for a wrongful act and imposing monetary penalties (with or without criminal charges) if the defendant is found guilty.

criminal law The type of law that pertains to determining whether a statute has been violated and, if so, imposing a punishment (fine and/or imprisonment) on the guilty party.

defendant The person or party in a lawsuit who is charged with breaking the law and harming the plaintiff.

due regard Appropriate consideration and responsibility shown for the safety of others.

gross negligence A more serious form of negligence that implies reckless conduct and a blatant disregard for the safety and lives of others. The line between negligence and gross negligence may need to be determined by a court.

liability Legal accountability or obligation.

negligence Failure to exercise due caution.

plaintiff The person or party who files a complaint in a lawsuit claiming to have been harmed by the defendant.

preponderance of the evidence A requirement in determining the guilt of a defendant that the majority of evidence presented in a case favor the plaintiff's argument.

preventable collision A collision in which the driver failed to do everything reasonable to prevent its occurrence.

reasonable doubt The lack of certainty that a person may justifiably feel based on the evidence at hand regarding the alleged guilt of a defendant.

true emergency A situation in which there is a high probability of death or serious injury to an individual or of significant property loss.

References

1. Auerbach, P. S., Morris, J. A., Phillips, J. B., Jr., et al. (1998). An analysis of ambulance accidents in Tennessee. *Journal of the American Medical Association, 258*, 1487–1490.
2. Clawson, J. J. (1991). Running "hot" and the case of Sharon Rose. *Journal of Emergency Medical Services, 16*(7), 11–13.
3. Colwell, J. J., Pons, P., Blanchet, J. H., et al. (1999). Claims against a paramedic ambulance service: A ten-year experience. *Journal of Emergency Medicine, 17*, 999–1002.
4. DeLorenzo, P. A., & Eilers, M. A. (1995). Lights and siren: A review of emergency vehicle warning systems. *Annals of Emergency Medicine, 20*(12), 1331–1335.

5. Elling, R. (1989). Dispelling myths on ambulance accidents. *Journal of Emergency Medical Services, 14*(7), 60–64.

6. Emergency Medical Response Task Force, for the National Association of EMS Physicians and the National Association of State EMS Directors. (1994). Use of warning lights and siren in emergency medical vehicle response and patient transport. *Prehospital Disaster Medicine, 9*, 133–136.

7. Garza, M. (1998). Ohio paramedic jailed in deaths from ambulance crash. *Journal of Emergency Medical Services, 21*(12), 21.

8. George, J. E., & Quattrone, M. S. (1991). Above all do no harm. *Emergency Medical Technician Legal Bulletin, 15*(4).

9. Hunt, R. C., Brown, L. H., Cabinum, E. S., et al. (1995). Is ambulance transport time with lights and sirens faster than without? *Annals of Emergency Medicine, 25*(4), 507–511.

10. NAEMSP. (1994). Use of warning lights and siren in emergency medical vehicle response and patient transport (Position Paper). *Prehospital and Disaster Medicine, 9*(2).

11. Pirrallo, R. G. (1994). Characteristics of fatal ambulance crashes during emergency and non-emergency operations. *EVS Monitor, 3*(4).

12. Slattery, D. E., & Silver, A. (2009). The hazards of providing care in emergency vehicles: An opportunity for reform. *Prehospital Emergency Care, 13*, 388–397.

CHAPTER 4

Maneuvering Your Vehicle

OBJECTIVES

4.1 Identify gross vehicle weight ratings for the five types of ambulances.

4.2 Explain how size and weight affect vehicle operation and control.

4.3 Understand how physical factors such as friction, gravity, inertia, and energy affect vehicle operation and performance.

4.4 Discuss concerns related to visibility and quality of ride.

4.5 Explain how road construction and shape affect vehicle control.

4.6 Calculate following distance and know how to maintain a safety cushion around the ambulance.

4.7 Outline the potential hazards and cautions for driving in inclement weather.

4.8 Outline safety considerations for specific vehicle maneuvers such as braking and stopping, negotiating curves and turns, changing lanes, backing, parking, and crossing intersections.

SCENARIO

When John left his supervisor's office, he was mad. His partner had complained that John's rough driving made it difficult for him to provide effective patient care in the ambulance, while John thought his ability to operate an emergency vehicle was just fine. After John cooled down, he recalled previous comments from his coworkers about his driving. He had written them off, assuming they were just the kind of normal banter that exists around the station. Now he realized that maybe people had been trying to subtly give him a message.

John went back to his supervisor and discussed the situation again. Although John had kept up with his continuing education and always attended in-service vehicle operator training sessions, together John and his supervisor decided that perhaps he needed a bit more specialized training to deal with this issue. John's supervisor made arrangements for him and his partner to use a nearby parking lot for a training session where they changed roles. John pretended to attend to a patient in the rear of the ambulance, while his partner drove. John's supervisor gave him several simple tasks to perform in the ambulance: taking a blood pressure, applying a dressing, and removing items from the cabinets.

John quickly realized that caring for a patient in a moving vehicle is not as easy as it seems. The abrupt changes in direction and sudden starts and stops greatly complicated his ability to care for the patient. He also noticed that the ambulance's design made it difficult to wear a seatbelt while performing these patient care activities.

With the help of his supervisor, John made arrangements to attend a local emergency vehicle operations course. The course covered many aspects of emergency vehicle operations, including local laws and regulations, vehicle dynamics, and a practical skills component in which each student had the opportunity to ride in an ambulance as a patient secured to a backboard. After this training, John was much more cautious about his operation of the vehicle, and eventually he was asked to help train new vehicle operators. John worked together with his supervisor to implement new and recurring training initiatives for his department.

1. Have you ever been in a similar situation? If so, how did you handle it?
2. Have you ever practiced being the patient during a transport while someone drove the ambulance as if it were a personal vehicle?
3. Do your supervisors track driving issues?

Types of Ambulances

The U.S. General Services Administration identifies minimum requirements for new ambulances that are fully built from the chassis up. These requirements are outlined in a document known as KKK-A-1822F, which describes ambulances that are authorized to display the Star of Life symbol FIGURE 4-1 . The document establishes minimum specifications, performance parameters, and essential criteria for ambulance design to provide standardization for ambulances that are constructed properly, that are maintained easily, and that function reliably.

There are five different types of ambulances, based on gross vehicle weight and design TABLE 4-1 . All vehicles have a **gross vehicle weight rating (GVWR)**, which represents the manufacturer's maximum allowable weight limit of the vehicle. On Star of Life ambulances, this rating is documented on a specification tag FIGURE 4-2 . It is illustrated by the letters GVWR and may be divided into front and rear axle weights, with a total vehicle weight illustrated. This total exemplifies the fact that neither the front nor the rear axle should be overloaded, and the complete

vehicle needs to fall within the GVWR. If it is exceeded, the manufacturer will not back the vehicle's warranty and the vehicle will not perform safely.

Type 1 ambulances have a GVWR of 10,001 to 14,000 pounds FIGURE 4-3A . The design is a cab chassis furnished with a modular ambulance body. This vehicle is designed with a replaceable

Figure 4-1 The Star of Life symbol demonstrates that a vehicle meets federal standards for quality performance.
Courtesy of the U.S. Department of Transportation, National Highway Traffic Safety Administration.

Table 4-1 Gross Vehicle Weight Ratings

Ambulance Type	Gross Vehicle Weight Rating (pounds)
Type 1 additional duty (AD)	> 14,001
Type 1	10,001 to 14,000
Type 2	9,201 to 10,000
Type 3	10,001 to 14,000
Type 3 AD	> 14,001

© Jones & Bartlett Learning.

CERTIFIED "STAR OF LIFE" AMBULANCE

MFG
BY _____

DATE OF
MANUFACTURE MO, YR_____

ADDRESS _____

CITY _____ STATE ___ ZIP _____

This Ambulance conforms to Federal Specification KKK-A-1822 in effect on the date of manufacture shown above.

AMBULANCE IDENTIFICATION NUMBER _____

TYPE - CLASS - FLOOR PLAN - SERIAL NO.

CURB WEIGHT	PAYLOAD MAX	GROSS WT. MAX
kg/lbs.	kg/lbs.	kg/lbs.

Figure 4-2 A sample label, featuring the GVWR, for a certified Star of Life ambulance.
Reproduced from the Federal Specification for the "Star-of-Life Ambulance," KKK-A-1822E.

Figure 4-3 A. Type 1 ambulance. **B.** Type 1 AD ambulance.
© Leonard Zhukovsky/Shutterstock. © imac/Alamy.

Figure 4-4 Type 2 ambulance.
© Osage Ambulances.

modular box for patient care. A small pass-through (a minimum size of 150 square inches) is required between the front of the patient module and the rear of the driver compartment. Type 1 additional duty (AD) ambulances have an increased GVWR of 14,001 pounds or more FIGURE 4-3B .

Type 2 ambulances have a GVWR of 9,201 to 10,000 pounds. They are standard long wheelbase vans that are customized to meet emergency vehicle and patient care specifications FIGURE 4-4 . They are typically designed with a raised roof to meet patient compartment requirements.

Type 3 ambulances have a GVWR of 10,001 to 14,000 pounds FIGURE 4-5A . The design is a cutaway van with an integrated modular body. This vehicle style has a required walk-through opening between the driver compartment and the patient module. If a door is included, it must have the 150-square-inch window at the driver's eye level. Type 3 AD ambulances have an increased GVWR of 14,001 pounds or more FIGURE 4-5B .

The term **payload** refers to the amount of weight the vehicle can carry within its GVWR ratings. The GVWR is the total permissible weight, which includes the weight of the vehicle, equipment, fuel, and personnel. For example, if the GVWR of the ambulance is 14,000 pounds and the empty vehicle weighs 11,000 pounds, no more than 3,000 pounds of equipment and personnel can be carried at any given time.

Figure 4-5 **A.** Type 3 ambulance. **B.** Type 3 AD ambulance.

© HHakim/iStock/Getty.   Courtesy of Cromwell Emergency Vehicles, Inc.

Figure 4-6 A 40,000-pound fire truck traveling at 20 mph has the same kinetic energy as a 10,000-pound ambulance traveling at 40 mph.

© Jones & Bartlett Learning.

Physical Factors Affecting Vehicle Operation and Performance

Several physical factors affect a vehicle's operation and performance. Friction is the resistance of one object to sliding over another. Soft, tacky materials have a higher degree of friction than hard, smooth materials. For example, rubber has more friction on asphalt than it does on wet ice. Gravity is the force that pulls objects toward the earth, resulting in what we know as weight. Weight gives the vehicle the ability to produce friction against a road surface.

Inertia is a moving object's resistance to change in its direction or speed. Inertia is affected by the weight of the object and the distribution of its weight. Additionally, inertia is affected by the speed of the vehicle. The slower the vehicle is moving, the more likely it is to resist a change of direction. A vehicle has two forms of energy, potential and kinetic. Potential energy is the energy the vehicle is capable of exerting, measured while at rest. Kinetic energy is the energy a moving vehicle has based on its weight and speed of travel FIGURE 4-6 . The formula

used to calculate kinetic energy (KE) is one half of the weight (or mass, m) multiplied by the speed (or velocity, v) squared. In mathematical terms, this equation is:

$$KE = \tfrac{1}{2}\, m \times v^2$$

What this formula tells us is that the speed has a much greater effect on kinetic energy than the vehicle's weight. Simply stated, doubling the vehicle's speed quadruples the kinetic energy (and its potential to cause damage if it were to collide with an object). This is why vehicle operators must be mindful of their speed. Driving just a little bit faster equates to a much greater stopping distance, difficulty in handling the vehicle, and increased impact force in the event of a collision.

Visibility

Ambulances typically have multiple mirrors mounted to increase the vehicle operator's field of vision around the vehicle. You should always ensure that these mirrors are properly adjusted. Also be aware that these mirrors may block the view across an intersection or roadway. Electronic mirrors, which are installed on some vehicles, make adjustment much easier for multiple drivers. Mirrors may also have a heating element to help remove snow and ice for increased visibility in inclement weather.

The use of convex mirrors is necessary to visualize blind spots on the sides of the ambulance. These mirrors give a wide field of vision, but they distort objects and make them appear farther away than they are FIGURE 4-7 . As a result, convex mirrors should be used with caution in judging distance, especially when backing or changing lanes.

It is also important to keep the driver's view of the mirrors clear. As mobile data computers or terminals are installed, it is important to make sure the terminal and its mounts do not block the driver's view of any mirror. These additional items in the cab can create blind spots and decrease the driver's view if not carefully installed.

Backup cameras are very useful for visualizing total blind spots, such as areas directly behind the vehicle FIGURE 4-8 . The technology now exists for a backup camera to share a screen with a global positioning system (GPS) unit so that the camera's image is displayed when the vehicle is in reverse. Some systems allow multiple camera heads to be utilized with one screen, and the vehicle operator can toggle back and forth between the cameras, visualizing the hazard at that particular time. The backup camera should never be used in lieu of a spotter, but rather in conjunction with the spotter for a more complete field of vision while backing.

Road Construction

To be in full control of the vehicle, you must also be aware of the driving environment. Road surfaces and shapes may affect the vehicle's traction. The main types of road surfaces are asphalt, concrete, dirt, and gravel. Each presents different potential hazards.

Asphalt is a petroleum-based product, which means that it may leech oils from its surface, resulting in a very slick surface in rainy conditions (especially when it first starts raining). In addition, asphalt repair is often accomplished by patching the surface with tar or additional asphalt to fill in low spots or cracks. Water can seep into asphalt cracks, freeze under the surface, and push up a portion of the asphalt, which results in rough roads and slick spots. When moving vehicles constantly pulverize the asphalt, potholes may result.

Concrete is typically one of the most durable road surfaces available. It is virtually incompressible, so it is commonly constructed with expansion joints, which give concrete roads a characteristic "thump, thump" feel when driving, because each slab may have settled differently in places in the roadbed.

On dirt and gravel roads, the emergency vehicle operator must make adjustments for a reduced amount of friction with the road surface. Stopping distances are increased on these types of roads because the surface promotes sliding between the road and the vehicle tires. In addition, like any other large, heavy vehicle, ambulances create flying bits of gravel that can be hazardous to other vehicles or pedestrians in the area and can create large dust clouds that reduce visibility. Whenever you are driving on these often-irregular road surfaces, you should be mindful of the vehicle's underbody clearance. Use caution to avoid large potholes or other irregularities that could cause the bottom of the ambulance to strike the road, causing significant damage to the vehicle.

Road shape is also an important consideration. Learning to read the road **contour** (curvature) can make you a much safer emergency vehicle operator. For example, noting the tree line in the distance can help alert you to upcoming curves. Roads have a **crown** (slope) to facilitate debris and water drainage from the surface. Although this is commonly a very gentle angle, on certain roadways it can relate to a large **camber** (arched surface, or road bank) and sometimes cause awkward vehicle handling FIGURE 4-9.

A road rises from the gutters to the crown of the road and slopes back downward toward the gutters. When a vehicle is on the road, the crown is most likely to the driver's left or just under

Figure 4-7 Contrasting views from a regular mirror (top) and a convex mirror (bottom).
© Jones & Bartlett Learning.

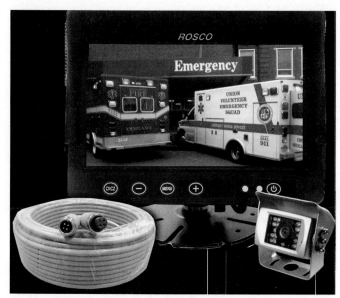

Figure 4-8 Backup cameras increase visibility into blind spots.
© Rosco Vision Systems.

Figure 4-9 The road's camber rises from the curb to the crown and falls back to the curb.
© Jones & Bartlett Learning.

the vehicle's left tires. The intersection of two crown roadways creates a valley at both the beginning and end of the intersection. When a vehicle travels through the intersection, its front wheels become airborne, and as they come down on the suspension the rear wheels simultaneously become airborne. This creates a see-saw motion from front to back that becomes more pronounced as the vehicle's speed increases. If a vehicle traverses the intersection too quickly, the vehicle operator could easily lose control.

SAFETY POINTER

While driving, pay close attention to details. The reflection of light off of phone and power lines can make you aware of these overhead hazards. Dark spots in the center of the driving lane may indicate oil drops, a potential slippery hazard.

SAFETY POINTER

Take special care on narrow roads not to drop a wheel off the road edge. If the vehicle does run off the roadway, remove your foot from the accelerator and steer it back onto the road slowly and gently as the vehicle slows down. Do not hit the brakes or turn the wheel forcefully to return the vehicle to the roadway, as doing so could lead to overcorrection and cause the vehicle to veer across the center line and possibly overturn.

Quality of the Ride

The biggest difference in operating an ambulance versus any other road vehicle is that you are transporting sick or injured patients. The emergency vehicle operator must find a safe balance between rapid transport to a medical facility and smooth driving for the patient and the provider providing care while en route. A good vehicle operator always considers the patient's condition. A conscious patient with a painful fracture may require extreme caution while crossing railroad tracks.

Remember that ongoing patient care is being provided in the rear of the ambulance. Taking time to maneuver the vehicle for a smooth, safe ride may increase travel time slightly but reduces the likelihood of a collision and allows for easier patient care and comfort during transport. Acceleration and deceleration are felt exponentially in the back of the unit versus in the driver compartment. This means that the operator needs to be conscious of the rate of acceleration during takeoff and deceleration during stops. The operator should also alert the crew if there will be any sudden change in speed, roughness of ride, or direction. The few seconds saved by rough, urgent transport will not likely make a difference in the patient's outcome and may place everyone in the vehicle in greater, unnecessary danger.

SAFETY POINTER

Emergency transportation should be carefully considered based on the patient's condition in accordance with local standard operating procedures and agency guidelines.

Safety Cushion

The emergency vehicle operator should understand and employ a **safety cushion** around the vehicle. This entails keeping a safe **following distance** from the vehicle in front, having an awareness of other vehicles or objects to the rear, and maintaining sufficient vehicle clearance on the sides of the vehicle.

To determine the correct following distance, you should take into account the total stopping distance of the vehicle, which includes perception distance, reaction distance, and braking distance. **Perception distance** is the amount of distance the vehicle travels during the time it takes for you to recognize a particular hazard. The average person takes one-half to two seconds to decide to stop versus making another move such as a lane change. **Reaction distance** is the distance the vehicle travels during your reaction to that hazard. **Braking distance** is the physical stopping distance of the vehicle with the brakes applied. For example, suppose a vehicle in front of you is slowing down. The perception distance would be the distance traveled while you turn your eyes to the road and perceive the hazard, the reaction distance would be the distance the vehicle travels from this moment of recognition until your foot presses on the brakes, and the braking distance would be the distance traveled from the time you press on the brakes to the moment the vehicle comes to a stop. TABLE 4-2 shows average distances traveled during perception and reaction time, as well as braking distances at various speeds and the overall stopping distances at these speeds. Remember, this table is for cars, not ambulances, which are heavier and require greater stopping distances. The table shows miles per hour as feet per second that the car is traveling.

For a general guideline, the following distance can be calculated by the **4-5-12 rule**. This rule recommends maintaining

Table 4-2 Calculating Following Distance

Miles per Hour	Feet per Second	Perception Reaction Distance (feet)	Braking Distance (feet)		Stopping Distance (feet)	
			Dry	Wet	Dry	Wet
20	29	44	19	24	63	68
30	44	66	43	55	109	121
40	59	88	76	97	164	185
50	73	110	119	152	229	262
55	81	121	144	183	265	304
60	88	132	171	218	303	350
65	95	143	201	256	344	399
70	103	154	233	297	387	451
75	110	165	268	341	433	506

Note: These distances assume a perception time of 1.5 seconds and a level asphalt surface. Be aware that these distances will be increased for emergency vehicles due to their larger size and weight.

Source: Modified from Oregon State Police—Patrol Division (https://www.oregon.gov/osp/PATROL/Pages/Safety-Tip---Following-Too-Close.aspx).

a 4-second interval between your vehicle and the vehicle ahead for speeds below 55 mph, increasing the interval to 5 seconds when traveling at speeds above 55 mph, and adding a 12-second visual lead time, which is to say that you should always be looking 12 seconds ahead for possible hazards and alternate travel paths.

In addition, you should be constantly scanning all of your mirrors and be aware of an escape route in case the vehicle in front of you stops abruptly. If you have nowhere to move to, you may need to increase the distance between you and the vehicle in front of you.

Inclement Weather

Weather conditions such as rain, ice, snow, fog, sun, and wind can change how you should maneuver your vehicle on the road. To increase safety in inclement weather, take the following steps. First, ensure maximum visibility by clearing the headlights, windshield, and mirrors of debris. If your mirrors are equipped with heaters, activating the heaters will help keep the mirrors clear of snow, ice, and condensation. Second, check that the soles of your footwear are clear of debris. It is important to recognize that heavy rain or snow boots may reduce tactile sensation and pedal control. Third, adjust your speed and stopping distance based on the road conditions.

Any kind of wet weather demands a gentler touch with the vehicle controls. Rain and snow lower visibility and require greater

SAFETY POINTER

On some vehicles with throttle and brake side by side, there is barely a quarter inch of clearance from the brake pedal when a large boot is placed squarely on the throttle. Be cautious not to allow your boots to get caught between these two pedals.

stopping distances. In inclement weather, you should drive slower than usual and keep in mind that you do not have the vehicular control you would under normal road conditions. Many states have laws regarding the use of headlights and windshield wipers during inclement weather. Headlights increase visibility and allow other drivers to see you. Windshield wipers ensure that you have a clear view ahead and should be operated at high enough speeds to clear the windshield of any unexpected splashes.

Wet weather can also affect the operation and efficiency of the vehicle's braking system. **Hydroplaning** can occur when a rolling tire rides up on a thin layer of water, thus preventing the tire tread from reaching the road surface. Most tread patterns on tires have small slits in the treads, called **sipes**, which allow water to seep up within the tread block so that the tire stays in contact with the road surface. The rotating tire sheds this water on each rotation. However, in severe wet weather or with very worn tires, the slits may not be able to empty, causing the tire to ride up on a layer of water (hydroplane), leading to reduced traction and directional control. It takes only one-sixteenth of an inch of water to hydroplane. If this happens, release the throttle pedal and allow the vehicle to slow down and sink back down to the road surface to regain traction. If you start to skid, depressing the brake pedal will increase your loss of control. If the rear of the vehicle starts to move to the left or the right, slightly steer into the skid to correct the vehicle's direction. You should always operate the vehicle at a safe speed to maintain traction with the road surface. It is important to note that traction is often more reduced when it first starts to rain. This is due to the mixing of oil from vehicles seeping up from the road and forming a slippery mixture with the rain. As the rains continue, that surface emulsion is eventually washed away and traction increases. Also stay alert for any pools of water, which if contacted, can cause the vehicle to suddenly pull in that direction.

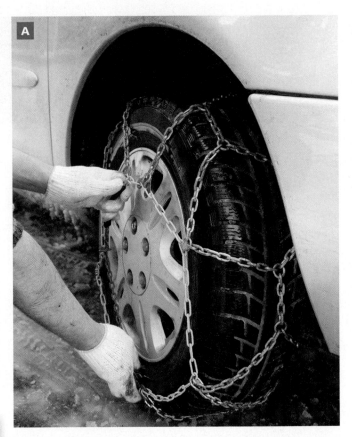

SAFETY POINTER

As part of your routine vehicle inspection, check headlights and windshield wipers. Discovering and replacing faulty lights and wipers during the inspection is much better than having them fail when they are needed most.

One of the most hazardous winter conditions is **black ice**, a thin, clear film of water that freezes on the road. Black ice typically occurs in shaded spots or on curvy roads in areas not warmed by the sun. It may catch drivers off guard, since it is difficult to detect and the rest of the road may be thawed. Bridges and any sections of road that are open below (such as those with a large drainage pipe under the road) may also present an unanticipated hazard, as cool air may freeze that section of the road when other areas may be clear.

In general, freshly fallen and unpacked snow provides a greater degree of traction than packed snow since the tire treads are able to sink down and bite into the surface of the snow. Depending on road conditions, it may be advantageous to drive out of the ruts and onto the unpacked snow surface. Remember that ruts can pull tires in directions that you may not want to go and will probably not match the width of an ambulance. Snow can also pack up around the headlights, emergency lights, and windshield wipers, reducing their effectiveness. Manual or automatic tire chains may be an effective tool for increasing vehicle handling on icy or snowy roads **FIGURE 4-10**.

Resting position

Working position

Figure 4-10 A. Manual tire chains. **B.** Automatic tire chains.

Automatic tire chains are controlled by the vehicle operator with a switch in the cab to allow for selective activation and are especially useful in areas where main roads are quickly cleared but rural roads may still be covered in snow and ice.

Foggy conditions occur when moist air exists over ground that is colder than the air temperature. These areas can be unpredictable and hazardous, reducing visibility. When driving in fog, slow down and stay oriented. Depth perception and shapes may be difficult to discern, causing a delay in reaction time to any potential hazards. Consider using windshield wipers to remove the thin layer of water that can develop undetected on the windshield. Heat on external mirrors can also be useful to reduce condensation. It may be necessary to reduce or prevent the use of emergency lights, since the lights reflecting off the fog may distract other motorists. In foggy conditions, use special fog or low beam headlights; high beam lights direct the light higher up, which increases the light reflection of the fog, potentially blinding the operator. Fog lights are mounted low on the vehicle and are designed with an amber lens to reduce reflectivity and penetrate fog **FIGURE 4-11**.

SAFETY POINTER

Be mindful that the effectiveness of audible warning devices will be adversely affected by fog.

Direct sunlight can also present a hazard by reducing vision. Use of sun visors can help. Squinting may reduce the brightness of the light but reduces your field of vision, so sunglasses are preferred. Be aware that bright sunlight can reduce your ability to see brake lights ahead, so you should increase following distances accordingly. Wind also poses a potential weather hazard, as most emergency vehicles are not

very aerodynamic. Vehicles with large, flat sides tend to catch crosswinds that can make vehicle handling difficult; slow down to reduce these effects. In areas subject to high wind speeds, it is often policy to remove ambulances from service when there are sustained winds of greater than 50 mph, and to deem wind speeds of 30–50 mph as conditions that will make driving the vehicle difficult to extremely dangerous. Finally, you may need to adjust your vehicle maneuvering to account for wet leaves and muck that can adhere to the road surface in the autumn and winter, creating an extremely slick surface at turns and intersections and potentially hiding underlying road hazards.

Unimproved Surfaces

Unimproved roads are those that are not paved, such as dirt or gravel roads. They are not limited to back roads in more rural areas and may be found in construction zones or in city parks after a heavy rain. Driving on unimproved roads raises certain considerations for the emergency vehicle operator.

Dry dirt roads have a loose top layer over a hard base that causes the vehicle to lose traction. Turning, cornering, and braking all become more difficult the faster the vehicle travels. Specifically, as the tires struggle to grip the loose dirt, the vehicle will tend to oversteer when turning and will travel a greater distance when braking. Further, ruts in the road can cause the bottom of the vehicle to hit the road and result in serious undercarriage damage to both the drivetrain and suspension, in addition to discomfort and exacerbated injuries for the patient during transport.

When traveling on a dry dirt road at higher speeds, the vehicle tends to kick up a cloud of dust behind it. This dust can be extremely dangerous because it creates poor visibility for other motorists or emergency vehicles. Keep the vehicle's speed down and check your mirrors often to ensure that you are not raising a cloud of dust. Communication is key when following another unit on these types of roads. Maintain radio contact in order to inform each other of potential hazards, and give instructions when needed. It is also important to increase your following distance. The combination of decreased visibility and diminished braking creates a dangerous scenario in which you have less visual notice of the need to stop, yet need a great distance to stop.

During the wet season, dirt roads become muddy roads, which can cause the vehicle to lose traction as it slides around on the slick mud. The mud may be so deep in some parts that vehicles can become stuck in a rut or mud hole and require a tow truck for assistance. Lead vehicles can potentially also throw a lot of mud out from their back tires, causing poor visibility for following vehicles.

Gravel roads have all of the issues mentioned for dirt roads plus an increased risk of kicking up stones that can damage other vehicles or injure pedestrians and bystanders. When following another vehicle on a gravel road, increase your following distance to ensure that flying stones and debris do not damage your windshield or other parts of the vehicle.

Figure 4-11 Fog lights can increase visibility in foggy weather.
© Osage Industries, Inc.

Agencies should have a policy in place that defines what roads, paths, or easements are permissible to drive on within their response areas. Remember that if you are in doubt about the condition of the road, stay off of it. You are of no use if your vehicle gets damaged or disabled while responding to help others. Emergency vehicles intended for use on unpaved or partly cleared roads should be specially designed to endure the rigors of that type of terrain, and the vehicle operator should receive additional training to ensure safe vehicle operation.

Specific Vehicle Maneuvers

As an emergency vehicle operator, you should be familiar with how to perform the following vehicle maneuvers and understand related safety considerations.

Braking and Stopping

In general, ambulances have a greater weight and higher center of gravity than typical motor vehicles and are therefore more susceptible to inertial forces when braking and slowing down. Slowing the vehicle can be achieved by decelerating with no braking forces (lifting your foot off of the accelerator and briefly coasting), though the operator will need to apply pressure on the brake gently as the vehicle comes to a halt to ensure a smooth and complete stop. In situations where you are cautiously allowing the vehicle to slow down but anticipate a potential hazard (e.g., if there are kids playing on the side of the street), you may choose to cover the brake pedal with your foot, but without applying pressure. This will allow a faster response if you need to apply the brakes to stop quickly.

Heavy use of the brakes can cause **brake fade**, in which the braking system overheats and reduces effectiveness of the braking system components. Brake fade is more common with heavy loads or during high-speed conditions. It is often the result of the brake shoes becoming overheated or the brake drum expanding to the point that the shoes lose contact with the drum. When brake fade occurs, braking action is ineffective and the stopping distance is increased. Some braking action may return after the system cools, but often the shoes, discs, or drums may be damaged and require repair or replacement.

Brake fade can also be caused by two-footed driving. Having even slight pressure constantly on the brake pedal, as during two-footed driving, will cause heating of the drum and can result in decreased stopping ability and unnecessary wear on the brakes.

Some drivers mistakenly think that in order to gain maximum stopping effectiveness they can apply pressure to the brakes and skid to a halt. However, sharp pressure on the brakes can actually increase stopping distances by forming small bits of rubber that act as ball bearings on the tires and reduce the traction with the road surface. Likewise, manually pumping hard on the brakes may be ineffective because of the intermittent loss of traction (skids) caused by sharp brake application. A better way to stop the vehicle in an emergency is to squeeze the brake pedal just shy of the point of the tire skidding. This provides maximum traction for stopping, yet maintains directional control. Most new vehicles have antilock brakes, which aid in brake control.

SAFETY POINTER

When stopping behind another vehicle, you should stay far enough behind so that you can see the vehicle's rear tires. This distance provides a safety cushion around the front of the vehicle and ensures that you can pull out if necessary.

Brakes are only one part of stopping. Tires must also be properly maintained because they are what actually grab the road and create traction. Rotating the tires is necessary to ensure tread wears evenly, which helps the vehicle maintain directional control. Uniform tread wear is just as important as proper tread depth when it comes to stopping. Without tires and brakes being in proper working order, controlled stopping will not happen.

SAFETY POINTER

Vehicle and tire manufacturers provide recommendations for tire tread depth. When you see damaged, worn, or bald (low tread) tires, it is your responsibility as the emergency vehicle operator to contact your maintenance team to evaluate the tires.

Negotiating Curves and Turns

Just as it does with braking and stopping, the high center of gravity in ambulances makes them susceptible to greater inertial forces when negotiating curves. According to Newton's first law of motion, an object will continue in the same direction and speed unless acted upon by an outside force. In the case of negotiating a curve, the driver steering the vehicle is the outside force and is attempting to change the direction of the vehicle. Centripetal ("center-seeking") force is also in play, pulling the vehicle inward and causing it to move in a curved path. Without this inward force, a vehicle will continue in a straight line. Friction acts as a centripetal force when negotiating a curve, and water reduces the friction between a vehicle's tires and the road surface. That is why the vehicle operator must take the same turn slower when the road is wet versus when it is dry.

Any reduction in speed by braking should be made prior to entering a curve. Continuing to brake while negotiating a curve can create problems with weight transfer. If the tires lock up in a turn, the vehicle will travel straight ahead, instead of in the direction that the wheels are turned. To safely negotiate curves, you should set an appropriate speed prior to entry, maintain steady speed throughout, and gently accelerate when exiting.

When turning, a vehicle will lean toward the outside of a corner. The amount of lean, or "roll," is proportionate to the inertia of the vehicle, which is affected by the speed and radius of the corner. Typically, slower cornering results in less inertia and less vehicle roll. Similar to curves, braking should be performed before entering a corner turn to set an appropriate speed. You should negotiate the corner at a steady speed then gradually accelerate while exiting the turn.

Different types of turns may require unique maneuvering. For example, typical roads are designed so that the camber causes a vehicle to lean to the left in a left-hand curve and to lean to the right in a right-hand curve. In off-camber curves, the vehicle leans away from the curve and is at an increased risk of overturning. Similarly, turns with a decreasing radius (one in which the curve becomes tighter as it progresses) may be very dangerous. In this situation, the speed set for entering the curve may be too fast for the latter part of the curve. Operators should pay special attention to ramp warning signs and their indicated speeds **FIGURE 4-12**.

Changing Lanes

Lane changes can be safely negotiated using the mnemonic **MOST**, which stands for:

- Mirror: Look for any obstructions in the mirrors.
- Over the shoulder: Look over the shoulder when applicable.
- Signal: Use your turning signals to alert others to your intentions.
- Turn: Safely negotiate the turn.

Following this procedure ensures that the area you wish to occupy in the lane is clear.

Special care should be taken when you are passing a vehicle on a two-lane road, as you will be crossing the center dotted line (not solid line) and traveling against traffic for a brief time. If it is necessary for the vehicle in front of you to pull off onto the shoulder of the road to allow your emergency vehicle to pass, you should ensure that it has a safe place to do so and that you can safely move around the yielding vehicle with an adequate field of vision. If there is nowhere for the vehicle to safely yield, do not force it to do so. Instead, keep a steady pace in the direction of travel and pass the vehicle when it becomes safe to do so.

You should be especially cautious when it is necessary to travel in an opposing lane to pass several vehicles. Be alert for any turning vehicles occupying this lane or any "leapfrog" passers (those who attempt to pass the yielding vehicles) **FIGURE 4-13**. Pass safely by indicating your intent by operating the emergency vehicle toward the leftmost portion of the lane. This shows intent to pass on the left and places your vehicle's headlights within view from the motorist's side and rearview mirrors. It also puts your warning lights in view for any oncoming traffic. Take care to avoid any hazards on this section of the road such as oil drip strips or taped road lines.

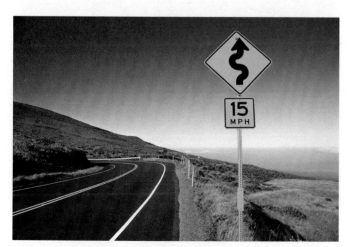
Figure 4-12 Pay attention to curve signage.
© iofoto/Shutterstock.

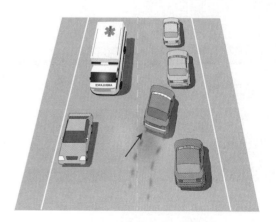
Figure 4-13 Leapfrog passers (arrow) make for hazardous driving conditions.
© Jones & Bartlett Learning.

Backing

Backing accounts for a significant number of emergency vehicle crashes due to the driver's reduced field of vision. To increase visibility, use a spotter and electronic aids, such as backing cameras. Spotters should stand to the left side of the vehicle and always remain in clear view of the vehicle operator. Hand signals should be prearranged, and you should roll down your window to hear the spotter's instructions or cautions FIGURE 4-14. Backing to the left or driver's side is usually safer than backing to the right, because the operator has a clear view out of the left window. If possible, it is best to back out of the traffic flow upon arrival, to avoid backing into traffic when leaving. It is

Figure 4-14 Spotter hand signals: **A.** Stop. **B.** Keep going. **C.** Left. **D.** Right.
Courtesy of Rob Raheb.

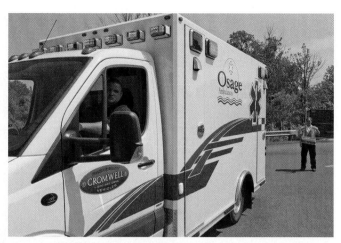

Figure 4-15 Backing safely is a learned skill.
© Jones & Bartlett Learning. Photographed by Glen E. Ellman.

much safer to pull into traffic with the advantage of full visibility from the front of the vehicle than to monitor traffic flow when backing out. When backing into a driveway or a single lane, it is easier to back with the road to your left where you have clear vision out of the left window FIGURE 4-15.

SAFETY POINTER

Tips for Backing

- Do not back the vehicle unless necessary, and even then, back only for the minimum distance necessary.
- Use a backup beeper (do not turn off automatic devices) or give a short blast on the horn before backing.
- Back toward the left if possible.
- Establish radio or visual contact with your spotter and keep your windows down so you can hear direction.
- Use a rearview camera, if available.

Parking

Perpendicular parking is a very common maneuver required of emergency vehicle operators in hospital bays and agency quarters. Perpendicular parking is usually easier if the vehicle is properly lined up with the space prior to the start of backing. This way the emergency vehicle operator can pick out visual cues, such as side walls or marking stripes to assist in positioning the vehicle.

Angled parking is similar to perpendicular parking. Many parking spaces in downtown areas are angled. It may be difficult to back out of an angled space, especially into a busy road, as an ambulance has more blind spots than a personal vehicle. Some downtown spots are angled so that the vehicle operator can pull past the spot and back in at an angle, and then pull out into traffic when leaving. It is best to pay attention to the angle of the spot and the amount of room available to maneuver before determining whether it is easier to back in or out of a spot. Either way, use extreme caution when backing into or against the flow of traffic.

When parking on a hill, consider which lane of travel offers the best vision of the blocked road. You may wish to place warning flares or cones to warn other vehicles of your vehicle's presence as they approach the hill. Alternatively, it may be necessary to use another emergency vehicle, such as a police car or fire truck, to block a lane of traffic to ensure safety.

Negotiating Intersections

Extreme caution should be exercised at all intersections, since this is where the most severe crashes occur. As a general rule, you should proceed as follows. First, check traffic to the left, since this traffic is closer and presents the most immediate threat. Be especially careful at blind intersections where your vision of oncoming traffic may be obstructed. Vehicle warning lights placed on the front corners of fenders may provide an early warning to crossing traffic.

If you are crossing an intersection with a traffic light, consider whether the light is fresh (recently changed to green) or stale (a light that has been green for a while). If the green light is fresh, you may wish to wait a moment before proceeding in case any late traffic entered the intersection from an opposing direction. When the green light is stale, you may not be able to anticipate when it will change to yellow. Therefore, you should determine a braking point at which you will have to make a decision to proceed through a yellow light or stop. If there is a significant amount of cross traffic waiting to proceed, this may be an indication that the light has not turned green recently.

When it is necessary to cross an intersection against a red light, you should first come to a complete stop at the limit line. Once you have determined that it is safe to proceed, you may approach each lane one at a time, clearing each lane individually as the intersection is crossed. Be careful not to force stopped vehicles into controlled intersections against opposing traffic. Left turns expose the vehicle to cross traffic for a greater time than right-hand turns do. When possible, position the vehicle in the closest lane available after the turn, and then complete a lane change if necessary. This approach avoids long sweeping turns where the vehicle crosses several lanes at once. It should be noted that due to the array of warning lights on the emergency vehicle, turn signals might be washed out during an emergency response. However, you should still signal your intentions. It may seem to be helpful at times to use arm signals to traverse across traffic; however in an emergency situation, you should keep both hands on the wheel.

A detailed discussion of negotiating intersections appears in Chapter 7.

WRAP-UP

Summary

- The U.S. General Services Administration's KKK-A-1822F identifies minimum requirements for new ambulances and outlines eligibility requirements for the Star of Life symbol, which provides specifications for ambulances that are constructed properly, that are maintained easily, and that function reliably.
- There are five different types of ambulances, based on gross vehicle weight and design.
- All vehicles have a gross vehicle weight rating that represents the manufacturer's maximum allowable weight limit of the vehicle.
- Physical factors such as friction, gravity, inertia, and energy affect a vehicle's operation and performance.
- Visibility can be increased by properly adjusting mirrors to minimize blind spots and using backup cameras and spotters.
- Various road surfaces (e.g., asphalt, concrete, dirt, and gravel) and road shape or contour may affect the vehicle's traction.
- Always remember that a smooth ride is important when transporting patients.
- An adequate safety cushion around the vehicle is essential, including a properly calculated following distance between you and the vehicle ahead of you.
- Use extra caution when driving in inclement weather conditions such as rain, ice, snow, fog, and wind.
- You should be familiar with your vehicle and how to safely decrease speed and come to a complete stop.
- When negotiating curves and turns, set an appropriate speed prior to entry, maintain a steady speed throughout, and gently accelerate when exiting.
- Use the MOST mnemonic to help you remember how to change lanes: *m*irror check, *o*ver your shoulder, *s*ignal your intentions, and *t*urn safely.
- When necessary to back the vehicle, use a spotter and back to the left, if possible.
- Perpendicular parking is usually easier if the vehicle is properly lined up with the space prior to the start of backing.
- Use caution when proceeding through intersections to avoid collisions with traffic from opposing directions.

Glossary

4-5-12 rule A recommendation to maintain a 4-second interval between your vehicle and the vehicle ahead for speeds below 55 mph, increasing the following distance to 5 seconds for traveling speeds above 55 mph, and encompassing a 12-second visual lead time.

black ice A thin film of water frozen on the road.

brake fade A condition in which brakes become ineffective secondary to heat buildup in the braking system.

braking distance The physical stopping distance of the vehicle once the brakes are applied.

camber The banking of the roadway; an arched road surface.

contour The curvature of a roadway.

crown The slope of a roadway, designed to facilitate drainage of water and debris.

following distance The distance between a vehicle and the vehicle ahead of it.

friction Resistance of an object to slide over another.

gravity A force that pulls objects toward the earth, resulting in what we know as weight.

gross vehicle weight rating (GVWR) The maximum allowable weight limit of a vehicle.

hydroplaning A driving situation in which a rolling tire rides up on a thin layer of water, preventing the tire tread from reaching the road surface.

inertia The resistance of an object to a change in its direction or speed.

kinetic energy The energy of a moving object based on weight and speed.

payload The total weight that a vehicle can carry within its gross vehicle weight rating.

perception distance The distance a vehicle travels during the time it takes to recognize a hazard.

potential energy The energy an object possesses while at rest.

reaction distance The distance a vehicle travels during reaction time after perceiving a hazard but before applying the brakes.

safety cushion An adequate vehicle clearance around all sides of the vehicle.

sipe A small slit in the tire tread that allows water to seep up within the tread block.

References

1. Oklahoma State Department of Health. EMS Statutes and Regulations. KKK-A-1822F. Retrieved from http://www.ok.gov/health2/documents/2009rulesandregs.pdf
2. Oregon State Police—Patrol Division. Safety tip—Following too close. Retrieved from http://www.oregon.gov/osp/PATROL/Pages/Safety-Tip—Following-Too-Close.aspx
3. U.S. Fire Administration, Federal Emergency Management Agency. (2014). *Emergency vehicle safety initiative*. FEMA FA-336. Retrieved from https://www.usfa.fema.gov/downloads/pdf/publications/fa_336.pdf
4. U.S. General Services Administration. (2007). *Federal specification for the star-of-life ambulance*. KKK-A-1822F. Retrieved from www.usfa.fema.gov/downloads/doc/DraftKKK-A-1822FCC.doc
5. WHIRL–Wind & Hurricane Impact Research Laboratory, Florida Institute of Technology. (2003). *Wind effects on emergency vehicles*. Melbourne, FL: Author. Retrieved from http://research.fit.edu/whirl/documents/doc_mgr/252/WindEffectsonEmergVehicle.pdf

Vehicle Inspection and Maintenance

OBJECTIVES

5.1 Explain the importance of vehicle inspection and preventive maintenance.

5.2 Demonstrate how to perform a complete vehicle inspection of the exterior and interior.

5.3 Explain the function, inspection, and maintenance procedures for the various mechanical components and systems of your emergency vehicle.

5.4 Explain how to respond appropriately to vehicle problems.

5.5 Discuss the value of road testing for vehicle performance.

5.6 Describe relevant standards and certification programs for vehicle inspection and maintenance.

SCENARIO

Kelsey moved the ambulance out of the bay for the morning checkout and noticed a pool of fluid on the bay floor. She noted the presence of fluid on her checkout sheet and reported the problem to her supervisor. The supervisor asked what color the fluid was, but Kelsey did not know. She returned to the bay area to look, but someone had already mopped the bay and cleaned up the fluid.

The supervisor explained that color is an important clue to determine what type of fluid is leaking. For example, motor oil is typically golden to black in color, antifreeze is typically green and watery, and transmission fluid is red with an oil-like consistency. By noting the color of the fluid, Kelsey would have been able to make an educated guess about potential vehicle problems.

1. Do you have a clear list of reasons for when and how an ambulance can be marked out for mechanical problems?
2. What are your standard operating procedures (SOPs) and training for checking the mechanical elements of the ambulance?
3. As an operator, what liability do you hold for the mechanical function of the ambulance?

Introduction

As the emergency vehicle operator, you are responsible for the proper mechanical operation of your vehicle. This does not mean that you need to be a mechanic, but you should have at least enough understanding of how the vehicle operates to identify potential problems before they occur. It is also important to understand your role and responsibility based on your department's policy. Each department will have different standards for which the emergency vehicle operator will be responsible.

Vehicle Inspection

Most emergency services require daily inspections of vehicles and equipment. Daily checks can help manage any known or developing problems with the vehicle by identifying trends as well as finding anything unexpected. Most services have a mandatory checklist that is completed on a routine basis FIGURE 5-1 . Never complete a vehicle inspection checklist without verifying each element on it. You should complete a thorough inspection of the entire vehicle prior to each shift to ensure there is no damage to the vehicle or any safety hazards that could affect the vehicle's performance. This inspection includes the vehicle's exterior, interior compartments, and the functional systems and mechanical components. As the operator of an emergency vehicle, it is your responsibility to be aware of the function, conduct an inspection, and perform maintenance of the various components of the vehicle for which you are responsible.

SAFETY POINTER

Vehicle inspection checklists are legal documents that can be subpoenaed, so take your documentation seriously.

SAFETY POINTER

During the vehicle inspection, emergency personnel should review the location and confirm the presence of all emergency equipment.

Exterior Inspection

All services want to present a professional appearance, and many people base opinions about a service simply on the appearance of the vehicle. Therefore, during the inspection, you should check that the vehicle body is clean and free of damage, noting any new damage that may not have been reported. Next, examine the tires to ensure they are in good condition and have adequate tread, with no bulges along the sidewall. Any uneven wear should be noted, and the spare tire (if present) should also be examined. The air pressure in the tires should be checked to

Daily Ambulance Inspection Checklist

AMBULANCE OPERATION	DRIVER-SIDE COMPARTMENTS	PASSENGER-SIDE COMPARTMENTS

Ambulance Equipment

Plugged in (electrical).............................. ___
Radio (operational).................................. ___
Telephone (operational).......................... ___
Emergency lights (operational)............... ___
Fuel (above ½ tank)................................ ___
Key (starts unit)..................................... ___
Tires (proper inflation, tread depth)........ ___
Inspection sticker (up to date)................ ___
Insurance card....................................... ___
IV warmer working (seasonal)................ ___
Windows clean.. ___
Unit clean (outside)................................ ___

Driver's Compartment

1–Hand light (6–12V).............................. ___
1–Spotlight (working).............................. ___
2–Protective gear (bunker coat, pants)...... ___
1–Emergency Response Guidebook......... ___
Driver's log book (mileage recorded)...... ___
Map/information book.............................. ___
Garage door opener............................... ___
Hospital map book.................................. ___
Keys/gas card... ___
Clean/trash removed............................... ___
Trip sheets box (with extra trip sheets)... ___
Completed patient paperwork/turned in.. ___
Accountability ring.................................. ___

DA Compartment (Oxygen)

1–Oxygen cylinder M (500 psi)................ ___
1–Regulator (2,500–2,550 psi)................ ___
2–Padded board splints (54")................... ___
2–Padded board splints (36")................... ___
2–Padded board splints (15")................... ___
Reeves stretcher..................................... ___
Scoop stretcher....................................... ___
1–Fire extinguisher (2A:10BC, charged).... ___
1–Folding litter.. ___

DB Compartment (Tool)

Bag buster... ___
2–Bunker helmets (hard hats).................. ___
2–Clear eye protection............................. ___
4–Disposable blankets (yellow)................ ___
Access Equipment Toolbox ...... # [   ]

DC Compartment (Drawer)

2–Leather work gloves............................. ___
3–Flares (30 min.)................................... ___
Tow strap.. ___
Battery jumper cables .... ___
Wheel simulator wrench .... ___
2–Goggles... ___

DD Compartment (VacuSplint)

1–SCBA/face mask (pressurized).............. ___
1–Vacu-splint mattress, with pump (child). ___
1–Vacu-splint mattress, with pump (child). ___
Vacu-splint kit (L, M, & S and pump)...... ___
Air-splint kit (6 pieces)........................... ___
1–Hand light (6–12V).............................. ___
Primary Trauma Bag.................. # [   ]

PD Compartment (Backboard)

2–Long backboards (straps)..................... ___
1–KED (adult).. ___
1–Pediatric immobilization board............. ___
1–Stair chair... ___

PC Compartment (C-Collar)

2–CID blocks (with straps)....................... ___

Cervical Collar Bag

1–C-spine collar (infant)........................... ___
2–C-spine collars (pediatric).................... ___
2–C-spine collars (no-neck)..................... ___
2–C-spine collars (short).......................... ___
1–C-spine collar (regular)........................ ___
1–C-spine collar (tall).............................. ___
– OR –
3–C-spine collars (adjustable).................. ___

PB Compartment (Side Door)

2–Oxygen cylinder D (> 500 psi)............. ___
1–Oxygen cylinder D (on cot)................... ___
2–Flowmeter (1–25 lpm) with guard.......... ___
1–Wrench (as required)............................ ___
1–Folding litter/cot.................................. ___
Unit clean/tidy (inside)............................ ___

PA Compartment (Drug Box)

1–Portable suction unit (& water)............. ___
1–Suction tubing...................................... ___
1–Rigid suction catheter.......................... ___
1–French suction catheter........................ ___
MAST with pump (adult)........................ ___
MAST with pump (child)........................ ___
Pediatric Kit.............................. # [   ]
Auto Vent Kit............................. # [   ]
Drug Box (locked).................... # [   ]

Jonesville VFC Ambulance • **111 Main Street** • **P.O. Box 978** • **Jonesville, MA 01803** • **(888) 555-1234**

Figure 5-1 The emergency vehicle operator needs to document that the vehicle and all its systems are in proper operating condition. Here is a sample page from a form used for this purpose.

make sure they are properly inflated. Remember that the proper inflation is determined by the vehicle manufacturer and not the tire manufacturer. Variations in tire inflation, such as a reduction of 3–4 psi (10%) can alter handling and fuel economy.

All external lights should be checked for proper operation, including emergency lights in responding and traffic-blocking modes. Check for signs of internal moisture and for rusted reflectors inside the lights, and also make sure the lights are securely fastened. To safely check emergency lights in the responding mode, it is necessary for the engine to be running with the transmission in park and the parking brake depressed. This will activate the high idle, which supports the power drain of the emergency lights. Next, put the transmission into drive with the parking brake engaged, and while one person has a foot on the brake, have another person walk around the vehicle to check for proper operation of each light, including turn signals.

Once the walk-around is complete, turn off all emergency lights, put the vehicle in park, and turn the engine off. Check that all doors open, close, and lock properly, including door locks on the patient compartment. Examine the windows; they should be clean and free of cracks and should open properly if designed to do so. The external antennas should be intact and secure. The exhaust system should be intact and directed toward the side or rear of the vehicle, as appropriate. The windshield should be clean and free of cracks and debris. The windshield wipers should include pliable wiping material that cleans the windshield without leaving any streaks. To check the windshield washer level, look at the reservoir inside the engine compartment. If the level appears low, add washer fluid to fill the reservoir according to company policy.

SAFETY POINTER

Antennas frequently strike overhead objects, so pay particular attention to their condition during the vehicle inspection.

Finally, as part of the exterior inspection, it is useful to check that all auxiliary equipment stored on the exterior of the vehicle is present and fully functional. Some outside compartment doors may not fully protect equipment from the elements, so steps must be taken to ensure cleanliness and regular maintenance of this equipment.

Interior Compartments

The operator compartment (or cab) should be clean and neat. Electrical loads should be switched off, and all radios, audible warning devices (e.g., public address systems and sirens), and other necessary equipment should be present, functional, and accessible. For example, you should check that fire extinguishers are placed appropriately in both the driver and patient compartments and that their expiration date and gauge levels are appropriate, that the nozzles or hoses are intact and free of obstructions,

that there is no rust or physical damage, and that the pins are intact and secure. It is essential for all equipment to be properly secured before the vehicle is in motion, as any unsecured equipment is likely to become a projectile and injure the patient or providers.

SAFETY POINTER

Equipment for basic maintenance, such as a tool set and jumper cables, should be kept on the vehicle. A basic set of tools may be used for basic repairs to the vehicle and may allow you to help someone else in need. Know your state guidelines regarding which hand tools are required to be on the unit.

Next, check that the seatbelt and restraints operate correctly without binding. All belt webbing should be intact with no cuts, and buckles should easily release when activated and close securely. Many emergency vehicles are equipped with air ride seats, which are adjustable for height, position, and angle. These seats should be adjusted for optimal comfort and vehicle control.

All mirrors should be properly adjusted for the maximum field of vision so that the vehicle operator can see down the length of the vehicle. Convex mirrors should be adjusted so the inside of the mirrors has the edge of the emergency vehicle as a reference. If the mirrors have a heat control, the operator should be familiar with this function. Examine the lights in the interior to ensure they are functional, and check for signs of internal moisture.

SAFETY POINTER

When mounting equipment, such as the mobile data computer inside the front compartment, be sure it will not block the operator's vision yet is within sight as needed.

The vehicle operator should also examine all gauges and meters to ensure they are fully functional and within an acceptable range for safe vehicle operation. The gauges and meters that should be checked are described as follows:

- The *fuel gauge* shows the amount of fuel in the tank. The vehicle should have an adequate level of fuel to respond to a call. If the vehicle has dual tanks, note which tank the gauge is reading and switch to the other tank to check the level in it as well. Experience with a particular vehicle will provide the operator with functional knowledge of its fuel range.
- The *oil pressure gauge* indicates the delivery pressure of lubricating oil to the engine.
- The *air pressure gauge* shows the amount of air in the air brake system. Typically, these systems have multiple

tanks with safety valves installed to prevent catastrophic loss of air. Many systems will have two different-colored indicator needles for front and rear pressure systems installed in a single gauge or multiple gauges.

- The *coolant temperature gauge* indicates the temperature of the engine coolant.
- The *speedometer* indicates the speed of the vehicle when moving.
- The *odometer* records miles traveled.
- The *hour meter* registers the number of hours the engine has been running.
- The *tachometer* registers the speed of the engine in rpm.
- The *voltmeter* (or ammeter) indicates battery voltage and shows if the alternator is charging the system.

Any warnings that are indicated should be reported as required by your company policy.

Mechanical Components and Systems

Your ambulance is a machine that is designed to perform specific functions. As with any other machine, it can be more efficiently operated and maintained if you understand its various mechanical components and systems. Ambulances have many of the same mechanical components as your personal vehicle plus some extras.

Engine

The power for operating the vehicle is provided by the **engine**, which in most cases runs on either gasoline or diesel. The engine creates power by combusting fuel in cylinders that are within the block (inner core) of the engine. This combustion process pushes pistons in each cylinder that are attached to a rotating crankshaft. The pressure of the combustion on the top of the piston pushes it down and the combination of all of the pistons moving in synchronization causes the crankshaft to rotate. Most ambulances have a tachometer gauge that tells the operator how many revolutions per minute (rpm) the crankshaft is turning—usually between about 500 and 3,000, depending on the vehicle.

The engine must have lubrication between the pistons and the cylinder walls to allow the pistons to move smoothly inside the cylinder. The engine oil, which is held in a pan at the bottom of the engine and is pumped through the engine as it is running, provides this lubrication. If the amount of engine oil gets too low, friction will build up between the pistons and the cylinder walls and may cause a piston to lock up inside the cylinder, ruining the engine.

The exhaust gases from the internal combustion are removed from each cylinder by the revolution of the crankshaft pushing the piston back up and the gases above the piston out through the open exhaust valve. These gases are routed through pipes located on the sides of the engine to the exhaust system underneath the vehicle. The exhaust system also includes catalytic converters that reduce the pollutants in the exhaust gases and mufflers that reduce the noise caused by the escaping gases.

The exhaust system gets very hot during operation and remains hot for quite a while after the engine is turned off. The engine exhaust gases contain carbon monoxide, which is a very deadly odorless gas when inhaled, so the vehicle should never be left running inside an enclosed area without adequate ventilation.

The internal combustion of the engine produces a significant amount of heat, which can also damage the engine. To avoid overheating, the engine has a cooling system that uses engine coolant to circulate around the outsides of the cylinders (within the engine block) absorbing the heat of the engine. This coolant is pumped through the engine and then through hoses to the radiator located in front of the engine. As the coolant flows through tubes inside the radiator, the air passing across the radiator around these tubes removes the heat it has absorbed from the engine. Once the heat has been removed, the coolant is again circulated through the engine to repeat the process. The coolant, which in most cases is a combination of water and other chemicals such as ethylene glycol, is very efficient at removing heat without freezing inside the engine if the outside temperature gets too cold and the engine is not running. The coolant often reaches temperatures in excess of 200°F during operation and creates pressures of around 15 to 20 pounds per square inch (psi) inside the cooling system. Most ambulances will have a gauge that indicates the temperature of the coolant. If the coolant temperature gets too high, the vehicle should be stopped and the engine turned off to prevent permanent engine damage due to overheating.

On the front of the engine, there are often several devices mounted that have pulleys on them. One or more rubber belts to the crankshaft of the engine attach these pulleys. This arrangement allows the rotation of the engine to drive these devices, such as an alternator for producing electricity for the vehicle, a power steering pump that provides hydraulic assistance for the steering of the vehicle, and an air-conditioning compressor that allows cool air to circulate through the unit in hot weather. In addition, on some units there may be an air compressor that provides compressed air if the vehicle is equipped with an air brake system. As you can imagine, if these belts break, the devices they operate will stop functioning, putting the unit out of service.

The engine compartment should be clean **FIGURE 5-2**. A clean compartment allows for the detection of new leaks or problems and helps the engine stay cool. Any belts should be intact and snug, with no cracks, cuts, or damage. Hoses should be properly attached and show no signs of leakage.

In the engine compartment, you should check the levels of oil and coolant.

To check the oil level, first ensure that the engine has been turned off for at least 5 minutes so that the oil reading will be accurate (oil distributes throughout the engine when it is running and then drains back into the oil pan). Next, locate the dipstick and remove it, wipe it off, and reinsert it. Completely reseat the dipstick and then remove it again and read the oil level in relation to the markings on the stick **FIGURE 5-3**. The engine dipstick typically has marking indicating whether the oil level is sufficient or additional oil needs to be added. Depending on the engine, anywhere from 1 quart to 1 gallon may be required to bring the level from low to full. When adding oil, ensure that it is the proper type and viscosity required for the engine of your

Figure 5-2 The symbols for coolant, transmission fluid, motor oil, power steering fluid, brake fluid, and windshield wiper fluid, and their respective locations in a typical ambulance engine compartment.

Photo: © Jones & Bartlett Learning. Brake Fluid Icon: © A Aleksii/Shutterstock. Motor Oil Icon: © Liudmyla Marykon/Shutterstock. Transmission, Power Steering, Windshield Wiper Fluid Icons: © Alexandr III/Shutterstock.

Figure 5-3 When performing an oil check, you must first wipe off and fully reseat the dipstick. You then **(A)** remove it a second time and **(B)** check the oil level.

© Jones & Bartlett Learning.

specific vehicle per the owner's manual. This information is also found on the oil fill cap of most new engines. If oil is leaking, you may notice pools of fluid under the engine in the color of the oil, which is typically golden or black. Conduct these checks and refill oil only if it is within your company's policy.

To check the coolant, ensure that the engine has been turned off for at least 5 minutes for safety. Removing the radiator cap when the engine is hot can easily release coolant as steam and cause a boilover of the coolant and possible injury. Most newer

SAFETY POINTER

Be knowledgeable about the engine of your vehicle and follow the manufacturer's recommendations for inspection and maintenance. This information can be found in the vehicle owner's manual.

vehicles have see-through coolant reservoirs with hot and cold markings, making it easy to visualize coolant levels and unnecessary to remove the radiator cap.

Electrical System

The electrical system provides all electrical energy for vehicle operation and takes on heavy demands in the modern emergency vehicle. Although efforts have been made through the federal specifications to limit the electrical demands of emergency vehicles, they are still heavy. There are several key components of the electrical system:

- **Alternators** produce current for the electrical system and are powered by an engine-driven belt.
- **Batteries** store electrical energy to help start the vehicle and provide a backup power source should the alternator fail; they typically provide only a few minutes of power under these circumstances.
- **Inverters** convert direct current (DC) power from the vehicle's electrical system to alternating current (AC) power—the same as household current—to enable the operation of hospital-type equipment, such as suction units, during transport or the ability to use an AC-powered accessory charger for charging cell phones in the ambulance.

Emergency vehicles typically have a high electrical demand and can occasionally suffer from electrical problems. Jumper cables may be useful to "jump-start" a vehicle when the battery has died. Care should be taken to clearly understand the procedure for jump-starting a vehicle, and eye protection should be worn when performing this task. Since jump-starting a vehicle can result in electrical spikes to the system, all electronic devices on the emergency vehicle should be turned off when performing the procedure. Always follow your service's SOPs, since some agencies do not allow crew members to perform any mechanical procedures on the vehicles.

Drivetrain

The drivetrain is the entire system of components that provide power to the wheels, including the transmission, transfer case, driveshafts, and differential.

The engine is connected to a transmission that is located behind the engine and that uses internal gears to convert the revolutions of the engine to slower revolutions that are required by the vehicle wheels as it is accelerating. As the speed of the vehicle increases or decreases, the transmission allows the revolutions of the wheels to change within the normal range of rpm of the engine by applying different gears. At slow speeds, a lower gear is used, and higher gears are applied as the vehicle reaches higher speeds. The transmission must have constant lubrication for the gears as well as for the internal hydraulics, which shift the gears when appropriate. Transmission fluid is a special type of hydraulic fluid. It is usually dark red in color and rarely causes problems unless a seal at one end of the transmission fails, allowing the fluid to leak out.

Most ambulances have automatic transmissions. New technology has allowed for the design of automatic transmissions to handle the heavier weight of emergency vehicles. These transmissions are hydraulic systems, which require proper lev-

els of fluid to function properly. Additionally, they are usually electronic, requiring a properly functioning electrical system to select the proper shift patterns.

Newer transmissions are being designed to utilize computer programming to prevent damage to the unit. For example, if the vehicle is rolling forward, the computer would ensure that the transmission would not shift into reverse before the vehicle was brought to a complete stop. Designs have also been developed to ensure that the vehicle cannot be placed into drive unless the vehicle is idling.

The transmission revolutions are transmitted to the wheels through a driveshaft and a rear-end gear that changes the direction of rotation and causes the wheels to turn. There are rarely any problems with this part of the drivetrain, but fluid leaking from the rear-end gear would be cause for concern. The rear-end gear is located in the middle of the rear axle (the shaft going from side to side between the rear wheels). If you find fluid (usually dark gray to black) leaking from this area, the unit should be put out of service for repair.

Routine preventive maintenance for the drivetrain includes checking transmission and power steering fluid levels. The transmission is a hydraulic system, and the dipstick is commonly marked with hot and cold notations. Some vehicles require checks with the transmission in neutral, and some in park, but almost always with the engine running. Make sure the parking brake is applied if the engine is in neutral. The procedure for checking the power steering fluid is the same as for the engine oil (just using a different dipstick and with the engine running). The power steering is also a hydraulic system. It is commonly checked with a dipstick installed on the cap and marked with hot and cold notations. The power steering fluid level should be checked with the engine off. Many power steering units simply use automatic transmission fluid, but make sure to follow the manufacturer's recommendations, found in the owner's manual and company policy.

Braking System

Historically, the braking system has been one of the most abused systems on an ambulance. Since most ambulances have a greater gross vehicle weight rating than a typical passenger car, these heavier vehicles are outfitted to handle additional stress and strain. Some vehicles are also equipped with auxiliary braking devices, which slow the vehicle by acting on the driveshaft, transmission, or engine. These devices normally act on the rear wheels and can be set to varying degrees of deceleration. However, caution should be used when using these devices on slick roads where they may cause the rear of the vehicle to skid.

There are several different types of brakes used in emergency vehicles. **Drum brakes** have a circular wheel hub with two semicircular brake shoes FIGURE 5-4. When the brake pedal is pressed, a piston spreads the brake shoes outward against the drum, using friction to slow the vehicle. Release of the brake pedal allows springs to return the brake shoes to their resting position. **Disc brakes** are designed with a disc and a brake caliper, with brake pads on the inside of the caliper FIGURE 5-5. The caliper is installed over the disc. Pressing on the brake pedal causes the caliper to compress the brake pads against the rotating disc, slowing the vehicle.

Hydraulic brakes use fluid to charge and activate the brakes. When you step on the brake pedal, fluid is compressed

Figure 5-4 Drum brakes.
© Toa55/iStock/Getty.

through the system and the pressure is applied to the brake pads or shoes, forcing them out against the rotor or drum. If fluid is lost due to a leak or other means, the system cannot pressurize and the result is complete brake failure.

Air brakes have the same task as hydraulic systems but function differently and require different maintenance. In a triple-valve air brake system, the air holds the brake pads away from the wheel, allowing it to turn freely. Depressing the brake pedal releases air from a chamber to activate the brake system instead of fluid pushing against the system. The parking system on air brakes also works differently from a hydraulic system. The park position on air brakes allows a mechanical spring to activate the brakes and holds the vehicle in place. This design enables a vehicle with common noncritical slow leaks in the air system to be parked for an indefinite amount of time. A certain amount of

Figure 5-5 Disc brakes.
© schlol/iStock/Getty.

air pressure, typically about 60 psi, is required to deactivate the spring system on the brakes. Their deactivation allows the parking brake to be released so the vehicle can roll. It is important to note that at any time while operating this type of vehicle, if the air pressure becomes lower than the spring pressure, the springs will take over, locking the brakes and causing the vehicle to skid to a stop.

Antilock brakes are a type of brake system that uses a computer system to detect wheel lockup and briefly reduce braking action to that particular wheel, allowing rotation and directional control to be maintained. Antilock brakes do not necessarily decrease stopping distance, but they protect the wheels from locking up and prevent the turning of the vehicle. Antilock brakes are especially useful on slippery surfaces. Caution should be exercised when using an antilock braking system on uneven roads, such as cobblestone or gravel, since braking distance can be increased.

Since inspection of the mechanical brake components requires the removal of the wheels, this process is not included in daily routine vehicle inspection. Brake systems should, however, be checked by qualified mechanics on a regular schedule. If the vehicle has hydraulic brakes, the brake fluid should be checked routinely. Most new vehicles are equipped with a see-through reservoir where the level of this fluid can be visualized. If the brake fluid level appears low, notify a supervisor. Low brake fluid usually indicates worn brakes, which will require the unit to be out of service for maintenance. Low brake fluid may also be caused by leaks, so make sure to check underneath the reservoir as well as behind each wheel for puddles of brake fluid. If you discover brake fluid leaks, this should also be reason to put the unit out of service. Never simply add fluid and continue driving the vehicle; doing so could lead to catastrophic brake failure. Some newer brake fluids are hydroscopic (absorb moisture), so opening the reservoir daily simply introduces unwanted moisture into the system. This problem can be avoided by simply looking through the reservoir to gauge the level of the brake fluid.

Air brakes should be tested daily by performing the ALSAPS method:

- *Air brake leakage test.* Depress the brake pedal and hold it. There should be an immediate reduction of air, but not more than 10 psi. Continue to depress the pedal for 1 minute. The system should not lose more than 2 psi in that time.
- *Low air warning test.* Turn on the power supply, but do not start the vehicle. Begin fanning (rapidly pressing and releasing) the brakes until pressure drops and the warning light and buzzer activate. Note that pressure on the gauge should be around 70 psi.
- *Spring brake test.* With the vehicle on level ground, push the parking brake in. Begin fanning the brake pedal until the parking brake "pops" out. Note that pressure on the gauge should be around 40 psi.
- *Air compressor cutoff test.* Start the engine and monitor the air compressor gauge. The air compressor should cut off around 125 psi. This process should be completed in under 2 minutes.
- *Parking brake test.* With the vehicle still running and the parking brake on, shift into gear and gently step on the accelerator, checking that the parking brake is holding.

- *Service brake test.* With the vehicle in drive and your foot on the brake, depress the parking brake and allow the vehicle to roll slowly 15 to 50 feet. Depress the brake and stop the vehicle. The service brake is functional.

If the brakes are used heavily during a trip, you may notice a burning smell coming from the area of the wheels. This odor is caused by the brake pad material overheating and is a sign that the brakes have been pushed to their limit. Occasionally under extremely heavy use, brakes can fail, resulting in an inability to stop the vehicle. This true emergency can often be avoided by limiting heavy use of the brakes through reasonable and careful driving.

Tires

Tires on the ambulance are expected to be durable and perform well at high speeds. They should be inspected at the beginning of each shift, and examined for proper inflation, adequate tread, and any signs of damage such as cuts, cracks, or uneven wear. You will need to check the tire inflation pressure to ensure that it falls within the manufacturer's recommendations for the specific vehicle type. These recommendations are normally located on a sticker inside the driver's door, the door jam, or the glove box door FIGURE 5-6 . Because the manufacturer recommendations for tire pressures are based on the gross vehicle weight rating, they may vary from the maximum pressure listed on the tire. It is important to follow the vehicle manufacturer's guidelines, while not exceeding the tire manufacturer's stated limits.

To check the tire pressure, you will need a high-quality tire pressure gauge. Tire pressure gauges come with different measurement ranges. Typical car gauges measure pressure up to only

Figure 5-7 Check tire pressure regularly.
© Jones & Bartlett Learning.

50 psi, but commercial vehicle gauges may have a range of greater than 100 psi. Make sure your gauge is appropriate for the task at hand. It is important to note that tire pressure increases when the tires are hot, so it is best to check tire pressure after the vehicle has been idle for at least 3 hours. To check the tire pressure, first remove the protective cap from the air valve, then firmly press the gauge inlet against the **valve stem** to prevent air loss FIGURE 5-7 . Read the measurement on the gauge and adjust air pressure as needed by adding air with an air compressor hose and nozzle or releasing excess air by compressing the needle inside the valve stem to remove air from the tire. Do *not* let air out of a tire that has just been driven or is hot; doing so can cause the tire to be under-inflated when it cools. Note, it should not usually be necessary to reduce the air pressure unless someone has previously over-inflated the tire. Make sure all tires are inflated equally. Unequal inflation will lead to poor vehicle handling as well as a higher likelihood of tire failure. Just remember that changes in weather and barometric pressure can change the pressure of a tire.

SAFETY TIP

Proper tire inflation is important to the safe handling of the emergency vehicle. Automatic tire pressure gauges will be included in those ambulances built or updated to meet NFPA 1917, *Standard for Automotive Ambulances.*

Figure 5-6 The tire pressure tag (inset) is typically found on the inside of the driver's door.
© Jones & Bartlett Learning.

Wear bars are small portions of rubber that lie underneath the tire's surface and perpendicular to the tread FIGURE 5-8 . As the tread slowly wears away, the wear bars become more prominent until they become level with the tire's tread. When this occurs, it is mandatory to change the tire since the sipes are not deep enough to channel away water. Actual tread depth measurements are tire specific, but commercial driver's license requirements of $2/_{32}$ inch can be used as a guideline. (For further information on treads, see the section on hydroplaning in Chapter 4.)

Figure 5-8 Prominent wear bars (inset) indicate that the tread is worn and that the tire must be replaced.
© algre/iStock/Getty.

Suspension System

The suspension system is what supports the vehicle above the drivetrain. Most ambulances are equipped with heavy-duty suspension systems to withstand the rigors of emergency use. Suspension systems have improved greatly in recent years, and many newer vehicles have air suspension systems that provide a smooth and comfortable ride. The suspension system in newer vehicles may also lower the rear of the vehicle to make it easier to get in and out of the patient compartment. Combined with stabilization systems, which reduce vehicle body roll (a tendency for the top of the vehicle to lean outward) in curves, improved suspension systems have made the vehicles much more comfortable and safer to use. Since the suspension system is all located under the vehicle, it should be inspected by qualified mechanics on a regular schedule.

Heating and Air-Conditioning System

In accordance with federal guidelines, all ambulances used to transport patients must have adequate heating and cooling systems to maintain a temperature of 68–78°F in the patient compartment. Most emergency vehicle heating systems work off of the vehicle coolant system. A series of hoses channel hot coolant to the patient module where a fan and radiator arrangement introduces heated air into the patient compartment. Electronic or mechanical valves controlled by a thermostat system regulate the temperature. Some vehicles are also equipped with electrical or mechanical valves under the hood that may cut off the flow of coolant to the patient module when it is not needed due to warm external temperatures. Most ambulance air-conditioning systems have one compressor and condenser to cool the cab and a secondary compressor and condenser system to cool the patient compartment.

SAFETY POINTER

While not required, it is a good idea to maintain a temperature of 68–78°F in the patient compartment so the area is at the proper temperature when the need to transport a patient arises.

Exhaust System

The exhaust system of the vehicle should be intact and functional, channeling all exhaust gases safely out the side or the rear of the vehicle. It is important to note where the exhaust exits the vehicle and to avoid aligning the exhaust output with the area of injured patients at a scene. Remember that the carbon monoxide in exhaust gases is colorless and odorless and can cause serious problems if it leaks into the ambulance. To avoid this situation, some ambulances are equipped with carbon monoxide detectors in the patient module. A qualified mechanic should regularly inspect the exhaust system, which is located underneath the unit.

OPERATOR INCIDENT

During the morning checkout, Danny was behind schedule and completed the inspection sheet in a hurry. Later that day, another EMT, Carl, was responding to a call and was unable to contact anyone on the radio. He had to resort to the unit's cell phone to get in touch with the hospital. After wheeling the patient into the hospital on the stretcher, he returned to the vehicle, but the engine would not start. He tried to turn the unit's headlights on to determine if there was a problem with the battery and discovered that the headlights weren't working either. He opened the hood of the unit and noticed the alternator belt lying beneath the radiator. The alternator belt could have been easily replaced if only Danny had done a thorough vehicle inspection.

Preventive Maintenance

Most EMS services require a daily inspection of the vehicle. This inspection is important to maintain the vehicle, helping it to last longer and perform more efficiently, and also to reduce potential liability from a failed vehicle due to a defective or damaged component. **Preventive maintenance**, regularly inspecting and servicing the vehicle, helps reduce equipment downtime and repair costs. It is more economical to schedule servicing and replacement at regular intervals than to pay for unexpected repairs. Preventive maintenance may be performed at intervals determined by the vehicle's mileage or a certain amount of time. For example, engine oil changes are not dependent on the vehicle's mileage as in personal vehicles, since emergency vehicles typically spend more time in idle (i.e., the engine is running, but this engine work is not registered by the odometer); however, tire inspection and maintenance should be based on the vehicle's mileage rather than a designated amount of time.

Maintenance schedules may vary based on the severity of the problem. Any problems that affect the safety of the vehicle (e.g., a cut in a tire or brake issues) should be addressed immediately. Less critical problems (e.g., a nonoperative clearance light) may be repaired during scheduled routine maintenance.

Road Performance

Some EMS systems include vehicle road performance in their required routine inspections, since certain problems can be detected only by driving the vehicle. If your service requires this test, you should check the following:

- The steering wheel should be properly aligned and should turn smoothly, accurately directing the vehicle with little play.
- There should be no unexpected noises. For example, a high-pitched squealing noise may indicate a worn or loose power steering belt.
- The brake pedal should be firm, and the vehicle should slow in proportion to pedal pressure.
- The brakes should stop the vehicle evenly without pulling to the left or right and should perform consistently, even during repeated stops.
- The vehicle should accelerate with smooth engine operation and no skipping.

Relevant Guidelines and Organizations

Several standards and organizations provide useful guidelines and resources for emergency vehicle inspection and maintenance. Vehicle operators should be familiar with NFPA 1071, *Standard for Emergency Vehicle Technician Professional Qualifications*. This standard outlines the minimum job performance requirements for a person qualified as an emergency vehicle technician who is engaged in the inspection, diagnosis, maintenance, repair, and testing of an emergency vehicle. While this standard is intended for the fire service, it does have some useful information that can be applied to all providers of emergency services. In addition, NFPA 1911, *Standard for the Inspection, Maintenance, Testing, and Retirement of In-Service Automotive Fire Apparatus*, provides minimum requirements for a preventive maintenance program for fire apparatus and sets a standard for many emergency providers and agency SOPs.

NFPA 1917, *Standard for Automotive Ambulances*, is becoming the new standard for ambulance design and construction and is steadily replacing the KKK specifications for ambulances built on or after January 1, 2013.

The Emergency Vehicle Technician (EVT) Certification Commission, Inc., is a nonprofit corporation that seeks to improve the quality of emergency vehicle service and repair. This organization offers a certification program for vehicle operators recognizing the training and experience they have in the service and repair of emergency vehicles. Automotive Service Excellence (ASE) is another nonprofit certification agency that tests professionals' vehicle repair and service abilities.

When your inspection or use of your emergency vehicle reveals a problem, you should report the problem in accordance with your chain of command and the SOPs within your agency. You should not drive a vehicle that you feel is unsafe. Remember that as the emergency vehicle operator, you will be held responsible for any collisions or injuries that occur. It is the employer's responsibility, in accordance with the Occupational Safety and Health Act, to provide a safe work environment, free of any hazards that may cause injury to the employee. States may have additional standards and different enforcement policies. NFPA 1911 allows the authority having jurisdiction to define defects considered unsafe for vehicle operation and outlines the responsibility to remove the vehicle from service.

WRAP-UP

Summary

- As the emergency vehicle operator, you are generally charged with making sure your unit is mechanically ready prior to your initial operation of the vehicle.
- You should be generally familiar with the mechanical operation of your vehicle and potential problems that might routinely occur.
- You should be very familiar with the daily inspection checklist for your vehicle and complete it in a thorough and responsible manner on every shift.
- You should be able to determine which maintenance you can reliably perform and which maintenance needs to be referred to a qualified mechanic, based on your company's policies.
- You should be able to road test a vehicle and handle any performance issues, including reporting them to the proper person.
- The emergency vehicle operator should mark out of service any unit he or she believes to be unsafe, pending repair.

Glossary

air brakes A braking system that uses air as a medium for applying the brakes.

alternator An electromechanical device that converts mechanical energy to electrical energy in the form of alternating current; automotive alternators use a set of rectifiers to convert alternating current to direct current to charge the vehicle batteries.

antilock brakes A computerized braking system that prevents wheel lockup, helping the vehicle maintain directional control.

battery A device that chemically stores electrical energy; it is generally used for starting the vehicle and short-term electrical use.

braking system The entire system that allows the vehicle operator to stop the vehicle by applying pressure to the vehicle's brake pedal.

disc brakes A braking system designed with a disc and a brake caliper installed over the disc.

drum brakes A braking system that has a circular wheel hub with two semicircular brake shoes installed inside.

electrical system The system that generates and maintains electrical energy required for vehicle operation as well as for patient care activities.

engine A device that provides the mechanical motive force for propelling a vehicle and powering its subsystems.

exhaust system The system for removing dangerous exhaust gases from the engine.

hydraulic brakes A braking system that uses fluid to charge and activate the brakes.

inverter An electrical device that converts direct current to alternating current; it provides 110-volt current.

preventive maintenance Scheduled servicing, inspection, or replacement of specific items in the vehicle to reduce potential problems.

suspension system The system that supports the vehicle and allows it to absorb the impact from bumpy roads without affecting the ride inside the cab and patient compartment.

transmission A device that provides speed and torque conversions from the engine to the wheels using gear ratios; it reduces the higher engine speed to the slower wheel speed, increasing torque in the process.

valve stem An opening to the valve that admits air to a tire and automatically closes to seal in pressure.

Additional Resources

Automotive Service Excellence, http://www.ase.com
Emergency Vehicle Technician Certification Commission, http://www
.evtcc.org

References

1. U.S. Fire Administration, Federal Emergency Management Agency. (2014). *Emergency vehicle safety initiative.* FEMA FA-336. Retrieved from https://www.usfa.fema.gov/downloads/pdf/publications/fa_336.pdf

Mental, Emotional, and Physical Preparedness

OBJECTIVES

6.1 Explain the importance of mental, emotional, and physical preparedness.

6.2 Discuss how avoiding distractions is a key component of safe vehicle operation.

6.3 Discuss how paying attention to detail helps ensure safe vehicle operation.

6.4 Outline the key elements of a safety-first attitude.

6.5 Discuss steps the emergency vehicle operator can take to ensure emotional preparedness, reducing the effects of stress and emotion.

6.6 Explain the importance of physical preparedness in emergency vehicle operation, including hearing and vision testing and hazards related to physical ailments, sleep deprivation, and medication and substance use.

SCENARIO

On Sunday, September 23, 2007, in Cranberry Township, Pennsylvania, the fog was so thick that it created virtual "white-out" conditions, making it nearly impossible to see the cars in front of one's vehicle or the headlights of oncoming traffic. An ambulance was transporting a 90-year-old patient for heart problems when it approached a standing red light. The emergency vehicle operator proceeded through the intersection with lights flashing, not engaging the siren until just 2 seconds before the ambulance broadsided a Chevy Cavalier with two occupants.

The patient, emergency vehicle operator, and medic in the ambulance all suffered minor injuries, while both the driver and passenger in the car were killed. The patient eventually died of a heart condition several days later, but it was not considered related to the collision. The roadway was shut down for 9 hours while police investigated the crash. Initial reports stated that the police did not know if speed played a part in the crash, but after additional investigation, they discovered that the emergency vehicle operator had been driving 70 mph in a 40-mph zone and had been under the influence of alcohol. The prosecutor stated that the patient's condition did not require the driver to exceed the speed limit. The emergency vehicle operator was charged with two counts of homicide by vehicle and two counts of homicide by vehicle while driving under the influence. She faced up to 14 years and 9 months behind bars but will spend 1 to 2 years in the county jail as part of her plea agreement.

1.   What would you do if you suspected a coworker of being unfit for duty?
2.   What conditions require emergency transport to the hospital?
3.   What happens to your visibility and the visibility of emergency lighting in the fog?

Sources: WPXI.com. (2007). Two Killed in Pennsylvania Ambulance Crash. Retrieved from http://www.emsworld.com/news/10339925/2-killed-in-pennsylvania-ambulance-crash; Kane, K. (2007). Ambulance driver charged in fatal crash will be fired under zero tolerance policy. *Pittsburgh Post-Gazette.* Retrieved from http://www.post-gazette.com/local/north/2007/11/11/Ambulance-driver-charged-in-fatal-crash-will-be-fired-under-zero-tolerance-policy/stories/200711110225.

Introduction

Every operator of an emergency vehicle is responsible for the safe operation of their vehicle as well as for the safety of the passengers, patients, and general public who might be affected by their vehicle's operation. Emergency vehicle operators must be mentally, emotionally, and physically prepared every time they get behind the wheel. Mental preparedness means having a safety-first attitude and concentrating on the details of driving. Emotional preparedness includes managing stress, anxiety, and other emotions. Physical preparedness includes avoiding driving when affected by illness or injury, undergoing regular hearing and vision testing, and maintaining adequate sleep. Obviously the use of any substance that can alter your body's ability to react quickly to an emergency should be avoided as well.

SAFETY POINTER

Emergency vehicle operators must ensure that they are mentally, physically, and emotionally prepared to focus on the high stress environment of vehicle operations.

Education, training, and experience are all important aspects of being a safe emergency vehicle operator; however, the most important aspect of being a safe operator is a personal commitment to safety and excellence. The concepts discussed in this chapter do not exist simply for the sake of creating company policy or guidelines. They must be embraced by the individual emergency vehicle operator. They play an integral part in ensuring the safe operation of an organization's vehicles and limiting the organization's risk.

Mental Preparedness

As an emergency vehicle operator, you must stay focused solely on the task of safely operating the emergency vehicle. The key to focus is avoiding distractions such as thoughts about what is going on in your personal life or technological distractions like cell phones or mobile data terminals. Many times the emergency vehicle operator is doing something in addition to driving. He or she is receiving urgent radio traffic or transmitting on the radio while navigating an intersection. At the same time, the vehicle operator and his or her partner are discussing the nature of the call based on dispatch information, and what equipment and potential additional resources they need. All things considered, the emergency vehicle operator is on scene mentally, but the vehicle has not even finished clearing the intersection.

One of the most prevalent mental distractions is mentally placing oneself at the scene while still responding. It is extremely dangerous and the emergency vehicle operator must instead refocus his or her attention on the present and the driving tasks at hand. Considering questions such as, "What equipment do I need?" and "What will we find?" can help responders mentally prepare but should not take precedence over the task of arriving at the scene safely. Failure to focus on vehicle operations can have deadly consequences.

Even during "routine" assignments, emergency vehicle operators must be mindful that simple conversations about "Where should I go for dinner?" or "What are you doing after work?" can lead to collisions. In the airline industry, pilots are required to have a "sterile" cockpit during critical phases of operation. This means that during critical phases of a flight such as ground operations, departure, or arrival, pilots are permitted to discuss only issues directly related to the task being performed. This approach increases awareness and decreases errors caused by inattention due to distraction. Research has demonstrated the effectiveness of the sterile cockpit, which can be adapted for use in a variety of settings, including EMS vehicle operation. The sterile cockpit is an important concept that should be embraced to help you perform your duties safely and effectively. Complacency is one of the EMS service's worst enemies. Remember, the smallest mistakes usually lead to the most horrific crashes.

Avoid Technological Distractions

Cellular phones, radios, and other technological devices are a major source of potential distraction. Many EMS systems rely on cell phones as the primary form of communication between the responding vehicle and receiving hospitals. However, cell phone and radio use distracts drivers and causes them to lose focus, leading to thousands of injuries and fatalities each year. When talking on a cell phone, the driver can be distracted mentally, emotionally, and physically, leading to tragic consequences. The use of cell phones by emergency vehicle operators in any form while driving is neither a safe nor an accepted practice. Some local municipalities and states have created laws prohibiting cell phone use while driving, and emergency vehicle operators need to be aware of and follow such laws. These laws can include prohibiting calls from supervisors, who should avoid calling crews while they are on calls *unless an absolute emergency*. If an emergency vehicle operator does use a cell phone during a response, the passenger should be the one to hold the phone to limit the likelihood of the driver becoming distracted.

The practice of texting while driving is especially unsafe and irresponsible. There is no way in which the operator of any vehicle can maintain constant visual contact with the road while texting FIGURE 6-1 . Even if you only take your eyes off the road for a fraction of a second, your vehicle is continuing to travel. At a speed of 55 mph, it will go 60 feet in just three-quarters of a second. Studies show that texting while

Figure 6-1 Texting while driving puts everyone at risk.
© Jones & Bartlett Learning.

operating an emergency vehicle increases the likelihood of a collision by a factor of 23 because it takes the hands, eyes, and mind off of driving. Distracted driving increases the amount of time it takes the vehicle operator to react and is a leading cause of collisions FIGURE 6-2 . There is simply no excuse for it. As an emergency vehicle operator, you must possess a safe and positive attitude and not engage in dangerous activities. You must aim to eliminate distractions and focus on the task of operating your vehicle safely.

Mobile data terminals (MDTs), which are becoming common in EMS vehicles, are intended to be used only by the occupant of the passenger seat or when the vehicle is safely stopped. Use of an MDT by an emergency vehicle operator while the vehicle is in motion is a dangerous distraction. Operation of this type of device requires the driver to remove one hand from the steering wheel and to divert his or her attention from the road. Focus on the screen and/or keyboard of the device takes the

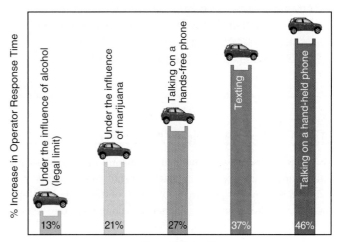

Figure 6-2 Driving distractions and their respective percentage increase on the operator's response time.
Data from Reed, N., and R. Robbins. "The Effect Of Text Messaging On Driver Behaviour: A Simulator Study." RAC Foundation. Transport Research Laboratory, 1 Sept. 2008. http://www.racfoundation.org.

driver's attention completely away from what is happening in front of and around the vehicle. It only takes a second of distraction for a collision to occur. For this reason, use of MDTs should be restricted by department policy as well as the individual driver's conscience. Coworkers in the passenger seat should be using mapping functions and using the MDT whenever possible. Drivers should plan their route before leaving a scene so they won't need to look at the map while driving, unless the vehicle is stopped.

Pay Attention to Detail

Paying attention to detail is a way of ensuring everyone's safety. As an emergency vehicle operator, you must ensure that everyone is properly restrained prior to moving the vehicle and during vehicle operations. You must be aware of your surroundings and environment at all times. Attend to the roadway environment and any hazards present, such as one-lane bridges, low underpasses, weight restrictions, narrow roads, or hazardous locations. Also pay close attention to your vehicle, constantly monitoring the dash, console, gauges, and warning lights. Lack of attention can create dangerous and unprofessional situations, such as driving with compartment doors unintentionally left open or partially open bay doors, leaving the garage with the shoreline still connected, driving with items or equipment left on rear bumpers or the hood, or overlooking hazards such as low wires, tree limbs, or overhangs. A quick walk around the vehicle prior to leaving is a good habit to avoid issues with open compartments and equipment misplacement.

Figure 6-3 Do not respond to aggressive drivers or let your emotions get the best of you.
© Jones & Bartlett Learning.

Another risky behavior is aggressive driving, which can stem from knowing that the patient is in urgent need of hospital care. Aggressive driving is not justified even in the most serious patient situations, since the time saved in transport is small, especially when compared to the increased risk of being involved in a collision. Remember that the driver needs to keep a clear mind and focus on driving, not on patient care. Without a smooth transport, patient care can suffer. Keeping a safety-first attitude will engender good defensive driving and help combat the urge to become aggressive **FIGURE 6-3**.

> ### SAFETY POINTER
>
> Adverse weather conditions can make it more difficult to identify potential hazards. When operating in adverse weather conditions, you must pay close attention to details and remain aware of your surroundings.

> ### SAFETY POINTER
>
> Your personal attitude toward safe vehicle operations is the single most important element in reducing emergency vehicle collisions. Your ability to recognize emotional responses and maintain a mature attitude in dealing with these temporary visceral reactions can save your life, and the lives of your partner, patients, and the public.

Have a Safety-First Attitude

Your attitude is a key component of mental preparedness for emergency vehicle operation. Having a safety-first attitude can help you be mentally prepared. Examples of this type of attitude include remaining calm at all times, making sure the vehicle is in safe operating condition before moving it, and constantly evaluating your driving to make sure you are doing things the safest way possible under the circumstances. Allowing yourself to be lulled into a false sense of confidence when driving with your lights and siren on can result in mistakes that can lead to a collision.

Having the right attitude also means not responding to other drivers who are showing signs of road rage. Road rage is thought to be responsible for thousands of collisions, resulting in injury or death each year. As an emergency vehicle operator, you are held to a higher standard and should not let your emotions control your actions. Do not respond to aggressors; always be courteous and remember that the vehicle you are operating is a billboard for your organization and profession. *Consider that everything you do is being filmed and could be on the Internet 2 minutes later.* Do not take other drivers' actions personally. For example, a driver who fails to yield the right-of-way may have a vehicle with a quiet cab or may freeze when approached by an emergency vehicle. The person's inappropriate response was purely accidental and did not reflect any disrespect for you or your profession.

Emotional Preparedness

Another important factor in emergency vehicle operation is emotion. Our emotions affect us strongly and can result in dangerous behavior if not properly controlled. Anger and hate can lead to aggressive driving, while love, grief, fear, and happiness can be dangerous if we allow them to distract us while driving. A lack of concentration due to these very strong emotions can easily lead to a collision in which people could be hurt or even killed. Controlling emotions is a very difficult task, but it is essential to maintaining focus on the primary duty of operating your vehicle safely.

Stress can also interfere with your ability to focus. EMS by definition is stressful, so knowing how to prevent stress from affecting your driving is critical. Every person deals with stress differently, and no one technique will work for everyone. In addition, different types of calls affect responders differently. Most of us are stressed when the patient is a child, but we may just as easily be overstressed if the patient reminds us of a loved one, such as a grandparent. The important point is to recognize when you are stressed and take action to prevent it from affecting your vehicle operation. Remember, that without a smooth and safe ride, very little care will happen during transport. Furthermore, if the ambulance does not make it to the scene and then hospital, no one will be helped.

Stress can cause physical symptoms such as headaches, increased blood pressure, back pain, or gastrointestinal distress. These physical symptoms of stress will also complicate vehicle operation. To deal with stress, you must first recognize it, and physical symptoms are sometimes the best clues. Other signs that you are stressed include rapid breathing, nervousness or shaking, and a strong urge to do everything as fast as possible. Probably the most effective way of dealing with stress for most people is to attempt conscious acts of relaxation. Deep breathing or slowly counting to 10 (or higher) before leaving the scene may allow you to reduce the stress that you may be experiencing from dealing with the patient's condition, which can help prevent the stress from affecting your driving. This technique may be needed before the run starts as well. Emergency vehicle operators must be able to leave whatever emotions they were experiencing before the run at the station.

When responding to what sounds like a serious call, it is easy to get excited and allow your adrenaline to push you to take risks, reasoning that you have to get there as fast as possible. You and your partner should remember that many calls are not as serious as they sound when dispatched. In addition, you should remember that risky behavior while responding to a scene will possibly save a minute or two, while exposing you to a greater chance of collision, which will then take even longer to get help to the patient and possibly cause injury to others. Managing stress is one of the most important things you can do to maintain your focus on driving and reach your destination safely.

Physical Preparedness

Physical preparedness is essential to the operation of an emergency vehicle. To be prepared physically, you must start by having regular physical exams, including hearing and vision tests. You must also be aware of any physical ailments you might have that could affect your driving and must make sure you are getting an adequate amount of sleep. Finally, avoiding any substances, especially drugs (even over-the-counter ones) and alcohol, which can affect your body's ability to function, is critical. The emergency vehicle operator needs to be in sufficient physical shape to operate the vehicle and keep the crew safe at all times. Remember, your job is one of the most important. Every person in the ambulance depends on you. Their lives are in your hands.

Hearing Testing

People often take their sense of hearing for granted and do things that can diminish their ability to hear such as listening to loud music. However, as an emergency vehicle operator, hearing is essential to ensuring your safety on the job. Your hearing can be compromised by colds, sinus problems, headaches, and exposure to loud noises, such as sirens and air horns. You need to recognize and be honest with yourself when these types of issues are affecting your ability to hear well.

Hearing loss is usually gradual and often difficult for people to recognize until it becomes severe. You should have your hearing checked annually to ensure that you have not unknowingly sustained hearing damage **FIGURE 6-4**. As mentioned, exposure to noises such as sirens can result in hearing loss, especially when the exposure occurs over a long course of time, as is sure to be the case for EMS professionals. Noise levels within the cab of an ambulance are of particular concern to emergency vehicle operators. Headsets may be needed to help keep noise exposure within Occupational Safety and Health Administration (OSHA) recommendations, which can be found in OSHA's General Industry Standards, Occupational Noise Exposure guideline (29 CFR 1910.95). The emergency vehicle operator needs to ensure that noise levels and use of headsets do not interfere with their ability to hear other emergency vehicles or outside warning devices and should consider a hearing conservation program as outlined in OSHA 29 CFR 1910.95(c).

If an emergency vehicle operator has hearing loss, hearing aids may provide great assistance. Hearing aids must be worn correctly, with the volume properly adjusted.

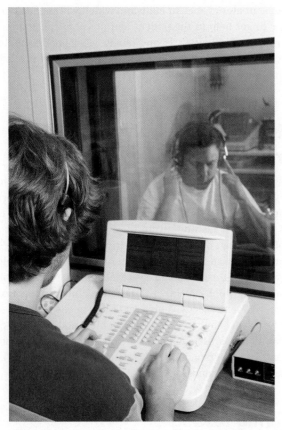

Figure 6-4 Annual hearing tests are essential to ensure your ability to perform your job safely.
© aabejon/iStock/Getty.

SAFETY POINTER

EMS leaders and personnel should ensure systems are in place to prevent hearing loss. The siren speaker should not be mounted directly over the front cab, and vehicle windows should be closed to minimize siren noise in the cab. Some services have also considered the use of ear protection.

SAFETY POINTER

Use of the siren and other audible warning devices may affect the emergency vehicle operator's hearing over time, thereby increasing the risk of vehicle collisions. Undergo regular hearing tests and take steps to protect your hearing.

Vision Testing

While it may seem obvious that a person should have good vision to safely operate an emergency vehicle, there are many people who drive every day with serious visual impairments. There are many conditions that affect a person's vision, including the following:

- Color blindness
- Night blindness
- Farsightedness (hyperopia)
- Nearsightedness (myopia)
- Eye irritation
- Age
- Medical conditions (e.g., colds or allergies)
- Incorrect eyeglass prescriptions
- Self-tinting eyeglass lenses
- Failure to get annual eye exams

It is important to recognize that vision changes. Annual eye exams are necessary to pick up on any changes in vision **FIGURE 6-5**. Some insurance policies cover the cost of annual eye exams, but they are necessary even if not covered by insurance. In addition, age plays a major role in your vision. It is quite common for a person to have a change in vision around 40 years of age. It is not adequate to rely solely on the eye exam given every several years to renew your driver's license as proof that

---

SAFETY POINTER

Some emergency vehicle operators wear contact lenses during the day and resort to glasses for calls during the night. This is fine, as long as they have the most up-to-date prescription.

Figure 6-5 You should get your vision checked every year.
© BSIP SA/Alamy.

your vision is acceptable. It is important to remember that if your driver's license says you are to wear corrective lenses, then they are required while operating the ambulance.

Physical Ailments

You must be aware of your body and sensitive to any health problems, injuries, or illnesses. While many people do not think that muscle strains affect their ability to operate a vehicle, these simple physical injuries can have a major impact on your ability to function. A muscle strain can significantly reduce your ability to move your feet, legs, hands, and arms, thus increasing the time it takes you to make sudden motions. In many cases, you will not realize how much your reaction time has been affected, and when an incident occurs that requires your quick reaction, you may not be able to react to avoid a collision.

In addition to muscle injuries, a person can be injured in a manner such that they are required to wear a walking cast or a joint immobilizer. These devices are designed to help a person heal by reducing the function of the injured area. The subsequent reduction in function places the individual in an unfit, and therefore unsafe, state to operate an emergency vehicle. When a person is required to wear any type of immobilizing device, he or she should not operate an emergency vehicle.

Illnesses such as colds, flu, gastrointestinal distress, or headaches can also affect your ability to operate an emergency vehicle. While you may think you are not affected by a cold or a minor case of the flu, symptoms of these conditions such as runny nose, sneezing, or coughing will definitely affect your ability to drive a vehicle safely. Thinking about these illnesses or discomforts can cause a mental distraction for the operator. In addition, medications to control the associated symptoms will often make you drowsy. *If a medicine has a warning that says do not operate machinery, it would be inappropriate to take the medicine while working as the emergency vehicle operator.* Gastrointestinal distress can be serious as well, since having a sudden bout of vomiting or diarrhea while driving could easily lead to a collision by taking the driver's mind and eyes off the road. Even something as seemingly minor as a headache can be serious if it suddenly becomes worse while you are driving, especially if you are experiencing sensitivity to light.

During any illness, you may be distracted mentally and more likely to react negatively or aggressively toward other drivers. Whenever you are suffering from an illness, you must ensure that it is not severe enough to impact your ability to operate an emergency vehicle. Failure to recognize when your ability to drive the ambulance is impaired can greatly increase your risk.

Tired Driving

Sleep deprivation can be a common cause of driver error FIGURE 6-6 . Since EMS providers often work long shifts, including through the night, they often do not get the 7 to 9 hours of sleep that most adults require. While the excitement of an emergency call may make us think we are alert, many symptoms of

Figure 6-6   Safe driving practices involve never driving while drowsy.
© Jones & Bartlett Learning.

sleep deprivation can occur even in these situations. Symptoms of sleep deprivation include:

- Confusion or difficulty focusing
- Yawning or rubbing of the eyes
- Weaving within one's lane of traffic or even crossing into another lane
- Impaired reaction time, judgment, and vision
- Decreased performance, vigilance, and motivation
- Increased moodiness and aggressive behaviors
- Problems with information processing and short-term memory

Long transfers of nonemergency patients can also lead to drowsiness for the emergency vehicle operator and even episodes of microsleeping.

Mircosleeping is basically a brief lapse of consciousness or awareness that occurs when someone momentarily enters a state of sleep. A person experiencing episodes of microsleep will experience head nodding, heavy eyelids, and periods of long blinks or seconds of the eyes being closed. Generally, microsleeping is thought to be the result of sleep deprivation, though microsleeping has been seen in non-sleep-deprived individuals during monotonous or boring tasks. There is little agreement on the best ways to identify and classify microsleep. In situations that demand constant alertness, such as driving a motor vehicle or working with heavy machinery, microsleeping can lead to critical mistakes—a problem that is worsened by the fact that people who experience microsleeping usually remain unaware of it.

Since the emergency vehicle operator is required to function with the safety of all in mind, it is essential to never drive when drowsy. Taking turns driving with your partner may be helpful, as may carrying on a conversation with your partner when you are both in the cab at the same time. If you feel you are operating the vehicle while drowsy, you should notify your partner and switch roles, if possible. If both you and your partner are extremely sleep deprived, you should consider notifying dispatch

OPERATOR INCIDENT

All providers have their own circadian rhythms and hormones that physiologically regulate their sleep and wake cycles. EMS offers several styles of shifts, and it is important for providers to find the shift that best accommodates their lifestyle. For example, one provider was working the day shift from 7:00 AM to 7:00 PM but did not want to get up in the morning and had trouble getting to work and being prepared for calls without several cups of coffee. The same employee moved to nightshift, which was from 7:00 PM to 7:00 AM and woke up regularly without an alarm clock, was active prior to going to work, and arrived at work ready to take calls. Even when the activities were similar after work and this person stayed up until 11:00 AM on nights and 11:00 PM on days, the employee functioned better on nights than on days.

Emergency vehicle operators should attempt to find shifts that fit their personal rhythms and needs. In many cases, maintaining an ideal sleep schedule is not easy or possible, but doing so will help ensure that the emergency vehicle operator has the necessary energy to function properly.

and asking about taking your unit out of service. It is much better to deal with the ramifications of this request than to be involved in a vehicle collision caused by drowsy driving. The bottom line is that you are responsible for having enough sleep before coming to work that you will be able to complete your shift without encountering problems relating to sleep. Studies show that being awake for 18 consecutive hours results in impairment equal to a blood alcohol concentration of 0.05%. Being awake for a full 24 hours produces impairment similar to a 0.096% blood alcohol concentration, which is legally drunk in all 50 states.

SAFETY POINTER

It is extremely important that EMS providers ensure the safety of themselves, partners, patients, passengers, and the public by being aware of the signs of sleep deprivation.

Medication or Substance Use

Occasionally, EMS providers will get sick, and it may be necessary to take medications that can affect their ability to perform their jobs. Before you take any over-the-counter medications, read the labels to ensure they will not compromise your ability to function, and never take any medication that warns of drowsiness and advises against operating machinery or motor vehicles. You should be aware of any potential synergistic effects with other medications or caffeine. Be sure to read and understand all warning labels and package inserts before taking any medication **FIGURE 6-7**. Be especially cautious with cold, allergy, pain, diet, or sleep medications.

SAFETY POINTER

Always read medication labels carefully and seek advice from your pharmacist prior to taking a new medication.

Sleep aids are available over the counter and come in many forms. Studies indicate that sleep aids can cause effects more severe than alcohol, hours after being taken. There are documented cases of what is known as "sleep driving" in which a person gets out of bed and drives without any memory of the event. EMS providers should never take any form of sleep aid while at work or prior to a shift. If you are prescribed a sleep aid, you should consult your physician to determine what the time frame is between using the medication and reporting for work.

Figure 6-7 Read labels carefully and avoid medications that can cause drowsiness.
© Wellford Tiller/Shutterstock.

Although the use of alcohol prior to or during a shift seems ludicrous to many EMS providers, there are some EMS providers who use alcohol and then operate emergency vehicles and provide patient care. Although this may seem more likely to be a problem with volunteer services, it occurs in paid EMS services as well. This behavior is unprofessional and dangerous to everyone involved. The federal blood alcohol limit for commercial drivers is 0.04%, but emergency vehicle operators follow local and state-specific regulations and are not subject to the federal transportation rules of other commercial transportation workers. Even before this level, alcohol can slow reaction time, impair vision, cause drowsiness, increase confidence, and impair a person's ability to function.

It is also important that employees are aware of, and employers have, policies that prohibit alcohol consumption for at least 8 hours prior to shift. These policies will help emergency vehicle operators be cognizant that alcohol takes time to be fully eliminated from the body before the start of the shift. Remember, conditions such as a hangover can decrease concentration, reaction time, and the ability to safely operate an emergency vehicle.

The use of illegal street or other recreational drugs is unacceptable in all forms and at all times by EMS providers. Drugs can greatly reduce your ability to think, react, and function. In some instances, EMS providers involved in incidents that resulted in patient and provider fatalities and criminal prosecutions were found to have used recreational drugs before or during their shift. Any attitude that promotes rationalizing this type of activity is unhealthy and unprofessional. The only attitude to have regarding any type of recreational drug use is an attitude of zero tolerance. With states starting to make recreational marijuana use legal, it is important that employees and employers have clear policies addressing the use of this drug FIGURE 6-8 .

It is your responsibility to be mentally, physically, and emotionally prepared every time you get behind the wheel of an emergency vehicle. You owe it to yourself, your partner, and the public.

Recreational and Medical Marijuana

Applicants for employment and volunteer opportunities should be aware of the City of Colorado Springs' current policies concerning the use of drugs or alcohol.

These policies have not been altered by Amendment 64 as it was not intended to require employers to permit marijuana use and it specifically states: "Nothing in this section is intended to require an employer to permit or accommodate the use, consumption, possession, transfer, display, transportation, sale or growing of marijuana in the workplace or to affect the ability of employers to have policies restricting the use of marijuana by employees." Colo. Const. art. XVIII, § 16(6)(a).

This language mirrors the Colorado Constitutional provision allowing medical marijuana which states: "Nothing in this section shall require any employer to accommodate the medical use of marijuana in any work place." Colo. Const. art. XVIII, § 14(10)(b).

Civilian Policy (Civilian PPM #39), Sworn Policy (Sworn PPM #35) and the Drug/Alcohol Procedures Manual outline the City's policies and remain in effect. Specifically, Drug/Alcohol Procedures Manual, Section II, includes:

- An employee is prohibited from the unlawful manufacture, distribution, dispensing, possession or use of a Controlled Substance in the workplace or on City property.
- An employee who reports to work under the influence of or whose performance is Impaired through the use of alcohol or drugs is subject to corrective action in accordance with City policies and procedures, up to and including termination.
- Marijuana is a prohibited drug in Schedule I of the Controlled Substances Act and it remains a violation of City policy for any employee to use marijuana.

Marijuana, whether it is used medically or recreationally, remains a violation of the Federal Controlled Substances Act, 21 U.S.C. §§ 801 et seq.

Figure 6-8 An example of a marijuana-use policy, from the Colorado Springs, Colorado, Fire Department.

WRAP-UP

Summary

- It is your responsibility to ensure you are mentally, emotionally, and physically prepared to complete all aspects of emergency vehicle operations.
- Mental preparedness includes a commitment to avoid distractions, pay attention to details, and put safety first.
- Distracted drivers pose a significant risk to other motorists.
- Emotional preparedness includes reducing stress and emotional distractions.
- The emergency vehicle operator must be physically capable of operating an emergency vehicle at all times.
- An individual's physical capabilities can be affected by a variety of issues, such as illness, injury, sleep deprivation, medication, or substance use.

Glossary

microsleeping A brief break with consciousness in which a person loses awareness of his or her surroundings and momentarily enters a state of sleep.

road rage Aggressive or angry behavior by a driver of a motor vehicle that may include rude gestures, verbal insults or threats, or unsafe driving.

sleep deprivation The state of having an insufficient amount of sleep.

References

1. McCallion, T. (2012). *Consider the dangers of shift work: It's important to have a fatigue management plan in place. Journal of Emergency Medical Services*. Retrieved from http://www.jems.com/article/emsinsider/consider-dangers-shift-work

2. U.S. Department of Transportation. (2009). *Driver distraction in commercial vehicle operations*. Retrieved from http://www.distraction.gov/downloads/pdfs/driver-distraction-commercial-vehicle-operations.pdf

Emergency Response

OBJECTIVES

7.1 Describe how to communicate with dispatch effectively and safely during an emergency response.

7.2 Recognize the importance of route selection to a smooth and safe response.

7.3 Describe how to use warning devices such as lights and siren appropriately.

7.4 Demonstrate roadway command for maneuvering around traffic.

7.5 Outline how to safely clear an intersection against a red light.

7.6 Explain how to transport patients safely and comfortably in emergency situations.

SCENARIO

Steve gets a call on a rainy spring day for a 4-year-old boy whose mother found him unresponsive, not breathing, and turning blue (cyanotic), near some small toys. He and his partner plan out the route, and then Steve turns on the vehicle's lights and siren in the vehicle and starts to head to the scene. After a few minutes, dispatch contacts the unit and tells them that the address has changed due to a poor-quality phone conversation. This means Steve has been traveling in the wrong direction for about three blocks. He turns the vehicle around and moves quickly down the block, clearing traffic to the right. As Steve approaches an intersection with a red light in his direction and traffic blocking the vehicle's path, he crosses left of center into lanes of oncoming traffic.

He looks around the intersection and identifies a truck moving toward the intersection from his left that is stopping to yield the right-of-way. He also notes a stopped car in the lane next to the truck and another car approaching from the right, both yielding the right-of-way. He determines, with his partner's help, that it is safe and proceeds through the middle of the intersection. Just as he is about to exit the intersection, an SUV cuts in front of his vehicle from the right. The ambulance strikes the vehicle, which spins around out of control and comes to rest on the other side of the intersection.

Several factors may have contributed to this collision. First, most EMS providers, no matter how long they have been in the field, have some anxiety when it comes to pediatric patients. It is important to pay attention to the road and not be distracted by emotions or thoughts about caring for the patient after arriving at the scene. Second, the fact that Steve had to redirect the vehicle after going the wrong direction may have increased his level of anxiety and sense of urgency, leading him to increase his driving speed. Third, Steve was too quick to determine that the intersection was safe to cross. He should have proceeded with caution through the entire intersection, constantly scanning to ensure that there were no oncoming vehicles and constantly asking for his partner's help with clearing the intersection.

1. Do you use a global positioning system (GPS) or computer mapping device? If so, who navigates?
2. Are there run types that create anxiety for you when they come in from dispatch?
3. Do you trust your partner to clear intersections for you?

Introduction

As an emergency vehicle operator, you will have to determine how to balance the need for safety and speed in responding to calls. In situations that are considered true emergencies (defined as those in which there is legitimate belief that life, limb, or property is in danger), it may be necessary to expedite your response within your department's policy. In emergency response situations, you will need to know how to communicate quickly and effectively with dispatch, select an appropriate route, use warning devices, and operate your vehicle safely to arrive at the scene as soon as practical.

Emergency Response
Communicating with Dispatch

When you receive information from dispatch, be sure to identify the call location and type. This information will allow you to plan your route and determine what equipment and resources will be necessary. Be aware that this information may not always be accurate; if the person calling EMS is distraught, lost, or confused, or has difficulty communicating, the information can be severely compromised. Whenever possible, it is best if communication between the unit and dispatch be made by another crew member, not the vehicle operator. When this is not possible, the emergency vehicle operator should use discretion as to when it is safe to transmit information. Thinking ahead about any upcoming changes in the driving environment (e.g., intersections or curves) will help you avoid a collision. Waiting until you clear the intersection or come out of the curve before transmitting may be the safest course of action.

Route Selection

When determining the route to respond to a call, you should consider unique situations posed by the time of day, the day of the week (i.e., weekends, weekdays, and holidays), weather, and location. For example, during early morning commutes, traffic traveling toward the center of town may be heavier than traffic moving in the opposite direction; during off-peak travel times, you may encounter road construction; and at night you must consider loss of visibility and traffic moving at higher speeds.

It is always best to know your route before leaving the station or the scene. If you use maps for directions, then you might look at the map and plan your entire route before the vehicle ever moves; however with mobile data terminals and GPS technology, a trip guided by your partner will be more effective. A short time spent planning your route before leaving may save you time and will certainly make your response safer. Even if you know your territory well, it is a good habit to look at the map or computer quickly before leaving to verify the route you have mentally prepared. If you are in unfamiliar territory (e.g., making a mutual aid response), you should be even more thorough in planning your route or use a GPS or computer mapping device. If you have a GPS device available to provide directions, take the time to enter the destination correctly before leaving or, better yet, have your partner program it. Ensure the route the device recommends is not compromised by construction, heavy traffic, or some other unforeseen local complication. Allowing the excitement of the call to lead you to leave without knowing your route will often backfire and end up costing you time in your response.

Use of Emergency Warning Devices

Warning devices such as lights and sirens are used to alert and inform traffic and pedestrians of an oncoming emergency vehicle in order to aid in clearing a safe path. Emergency warning devices should be used whenever you are taking advantage of a traffic exemption, such as driving through a red light or traveling against traffic on a one-way street. When you use your lights and siren, depending on state law, you are to be given the right-of-way, but there is no guarantee that you will receive it. While you should understand how to use warning devices appropriately, you should not assume that they will be effective. Car manufacturers are competing to create a quieter interior, which means they are blocking your siren sounds. If a motorist or pedestrian does not yield the right-of-way, you don't have it, even though they are violating the law! It is your responsibility to stay alert, observe traffic and pedestrians, and operate your vehicle appropriately. You should always drive with caution and due regard for the safety of others.

There are several different types of warning lights and sirens that may be used in an emergency response. Lights come in a variety of displays and colors, and sirens provide a variety of alerting sounds. Your state and local laws, as well as your company policies, will determine the type of devices required.

Lights

Emergency lights are critical for emergency responses. While sirens are important for getting the attention of drivers near your emergency vehicle, emergency lights can usually be recognized from a greater distance and allow drivers more time to adjust to your approach. There are many types of emergency lights, and each has its advantages. Understanding the applications of these lights is important to the emergency response. Some of the types of emergency lights include the following:

- *On–off blinking red lights* are often placed on the upper corners at the front and back of the patient compartment. They are probably the oldest type of emergency lights still in use. When these lights are operating, one side will be on while the other is off, which creates an alternating blinking from right to left and vice versa, which will attract attention.
- *Light bars* contain different colors of rotating lights mounted on a bar and are usually encased in a clear hard-plastic protective covering. New models have

flashing LED lights instead of rotating lights. These light bars are generally mounted on the cabs of the unit, but they may also be mounted on top of the patient compartment. The bars usually include red and white lights, although in some locations they may include blue and/or green lights as well, depending on state, local, and department policy.

- *Strobe lights* are generally very high-intensity lights (usually white) that flash on and off very quickly, at a rate of several times per second. Because of the extreme brightness and the rapid rate of flashing, these lights can be seen from a significant distance, often much farther than any of the other lights. It is important to note that the strobes can be associated with causing seizures in epileptic patients and may need to be shut down when arriving on those scenes. The use of strobe lights should be used in conjunction with other incandescent warning lights, due to the fact that strobe lighting does not leave a lighting trail and can create a confusing setting for other motorist.

Most ambulances have a combination of these types of lights, and in many cases they are used simultaneously. Often when arriving on scene, the emergency vehicle operator may choose to turn off the strobes and the light bars but leave on the red flashing lights just to alert approaching traffic of the unit's presence. These lights, especially strobes, can create vision problems at night for other traffic as well as workers operating on the scene. When driving in foggy conditions, the emergency vehicle operator should turn off any strobe lights because they will reflect back and effectively blind the operator at a time when good vision is critical. Each state, locality, and department will have its own rules regarding which emergency warning devices must be activated. Often, emergency vehicle operators will choose to operate in emergency mode with lights only and no sirens. This is a very dangerous action that might be acceptable in a few situations, such as when traveling slowly through a subdivision very late at night when there is essentially no other traffic. The best procedure, however, is to use lights and sirens together, which gives you the best chance of being recognized so that others will move out of your way.

It is also important to note that some states have opted to have a flashing blue light on the rear of the vehicle to help traffic identify the emergency vehicle from behind as they approach it. Many states have similarly adopted a yellow or amber light on the rear of the vehicle as a familiar warning to motorists. Another change to increase visibility is the addition of reflective paint schemes or chevrons on the rear of vehicles. This feature will be further covered in Chapter 8.

Many states have also adopted "move-over laws" that require vehicles to move over or slow down when traveling in the lane adjacent to a stopped emergency vehicle with its emergency lights activated. It is important to be familiar with these laws and to understand that just because it is the law does not mean that all drivers will comply.

Sirens

There are several different types of sirens and siren sounds for emergency vehicle use. All sirens must meet a federal Department of Transportation (DOT) specification of 90–120 decibels as well as any local ordinances regarding decibel levels. Common siren sounds include the following:

- A **wail** is a continuous, repeating tone that modulates from a high to a low frequency and is generally used while traveling down a road or street.
- A **Federal Q** is a well-known and distinctive type of wail siren that is trademarked by Federal Signal Corporation. Traditionally, this is a mechanical siren requiring a brake to stop, but an electronic version is now available.
- A **yelp** consists of short bursts of modulated sound; this sound is generally used to clear traffic before entering an intersection or when traffic patterns become more congested.
- A **high–low frequency siren** repeats a high tone with a quick drop to the low range. This siren is used primarily in Europe; many motorists in the United States are not familiar with it, so it should be used only when a change of pattern is necessary to gain the attention of another motorist. Note that some states have banned this siren on vehicles and have adopted it as a civil emergency warning tone.
- A **phaser** sounds like a ray gun sound effect and may be used as an alternative to the yelp sound to clear traffic, though it is less effective. The phaser sound has a higher frequency range and has less sound penetration into traffic. It is a deceptively useless sound. The crew inside the cab hear a loud phaser sound, while the traffic around them hears nearly nothing.
- A **low-frequency siren**, or Rumbler®, has the ability to interact with preexisting sirens, providing secondary, low-frequency duplicate tones that can shake solid materials so that motorists and pedestrians may feel the sound waves and see their effects in nearby objects such as rearview mirrors. This siren type is effective in heavily congested urban areas.

Sirens tend to become **omnidirectional** (projecting in all directions) when their sound waves bounce off of other objects such as buildings and other vehicles, thus making it difficult to determine the exact direction of the siren's location. When a **unidirectional** (projecting in one direction) warning device is needed to help motorists and pedestrians identify your vehicle's location quickly, **air horns** may be useful. Air horns can be either electronic or pneumatic and are most commonly used in short, intermittent bursts. When used continuously, air horns can become omnidirectional and drown out siren sounds. Excessive use of the pneumatic air horn may also decrease the effectiveness of air-assisted brake systems.

In general, when using the yelp or phaser siren to clear traffic, you should engage the siren approximately 150 to 200 feet before the intersection. These sounds may be more effective when used in conjunction with the wail signal. No matter which siren is used, make sure to vary the sound when approaching and moving through the intersection.

your state's move-over laws because some require motorists to go to the nearest curb and others require them to pull to the right of their present lane.

You are expected to understand basic roadway signage and striping along with traffic control devices and the laws that govern them.

Regardless of which sound or audible warning device is used, it is important to know the limits of these devices. Most sirens are effective only 230 feet ahead of the vehicle. The faster your vehicle is traveling, the less time motorists and pedestrians have to hear and respond to the warning FIGURE 7-1 . If the ambulance is traveling above 40 mph, others may not hear your warning sirens in time to react. You should never assume that your siren will be heard by anyone, especially as car makers continue to develop quieter cabs.

When operating an emergency vehicle on a multilane unidirectional (one-way) road or those divided by medians, it is best to be in the middle lane or center of the road. This position allows traffic to pull to either the right or left to get out of the path of the emergency vehicle FIGURE 7-3 . On multilane highways, it is best to maintain your position in the left lane and move traffic toward the right. If traffic is extremely congested and is at a standstill, traveling in the center lane will allow traffic to clear a path more quickly by moving into the outside lanes and shoulder of the roadway.

Roadway Command

Vehicle placement on the roadway conveys your intentions to other motorists. When you are traveling on a multilane and bidirectional (two-way) roadway, you should position your vehicle as close to the center line as possible without crossing it FIGURE 7-2 . This allows you the most room to maneuver safely around stopped traffic. Staying close to the center line also avoids hazards such as double-parked cars, pedestrians stepping off curbs, people getting in or out of parked cars, or traffic moving to the right to yield the right-of-way. It is important to know

Traffic law exemptions are permitted during perceived true emergencies, but you are still required to use due regard and give proper notice of approach at all times. The use of an exemption does not grant immunity if you are involved in a collision.

Traveling at 60 mph = siren projects approximately 6.5 feet
Traveling at 30 mph = siren projects approximately 20 feet

Figure 7-1 At faster speeds, the siren projects a shorter distance from the vehicle.
Courtesy of FAAC, Inc.

Figure 7-2 On a multidirectional road, you should stay near the center line without crossing it to allow traffic to move safely out of the way and give you room to maneuver.
Courtesy of FAAC, Inc.

Figure 7-3 On a unidirectional road, you can travel in the center of the road to allow traffic to move in either direction.
Courtesy of FAAC, Inc.

When heavy traffic conditions will not allow you to travel with the flow of traffic, you may need to make a traffic law exemption and cross over the double yellow line into oncoming traffic. This maneuver is known as **moving left of center** FIGURE 7-4 . There are several important considerations you should take when moving left of center to ensure the safety of your crew and the surrounding traffic. First make sure it is acceptable by state law and company policy. It is always important to maintain a heightened level of awareness for any motorists who are not paying attention and are unaware of your vehicle's presence. Therefore, you should slow down, traveling at no more than 15 or 20 mph, and use your turn signals to notify people of your intentions. When driving against the direction of traffic, you should make

Figure 7-4 Perception distance is the distance you travel when realizing that you need to brake. **A.** This distance is increased when an emergency vehicle remains in its proper travel lane. **B.** When moving left of center through an intersection, perception distance is greatly reduced.
Courtesy of FAAC, Inc.

sure that oncoming drivers are yielding the right-of-way and are moving to their right, leaving the lane closest to the center line to you. Always remain vigilant for any motorists in the left turning lane (on your right side) who may attempt to turn into your path. As soon as it is possible to do so, move back into the proper lanes of travel. If the roadway has a median, you should not attempt to cross it.

SAFETY POINTER

Remember that traffic law exemptions are permitted only for the time that they are necessary and when allowed by state law and company policies.

Special Considerations

The preceding information is important on all responses, but there are other responses that will require special considerations. These include multiple-casualty incidents, hazardous materials response, and any type of technical rescue. These incidents generate a large response, with many emergency vehicles responding to the same location. Emergency vehicle operators need to be aware of this increased traffic and pay special attention to avoid collisions with other units. It is important to make sure intersections are clear and all vehicles are aware of which vehicles are going first and that they know not to proceed until all emergency vehicles have cleared the intersection.

It is also important to pay attention to special directions when responding to these types of incidents. Ambulances may be asked to go to a staging area away from the incident or a new location as the incident progresses. Preplanned routes may have to be adapted, and it is important that the emergency vehicle operator stays focused on driving and the passenger focuses on the new information, responding to radio traffic, and navigating the ambulance. These new instructions could be lifesaving, especially in hazardous materials situations where chemicals may be moving.

Intersection Analysis

One of the most dangerous maneuvers an emergency vehicle operator performs is crossing an intersection against the light. Intersection collisions frequently cause more damage, injuries, and fatalities than any other collision. Use extreme caution when taking advantage of this traffic law exemption. Be alert to any oncoming traffic, crossing traffic, and nearby pedestrians.

The safest way to cross an intersection against the light is as follows. Note that the steps involved are illustrated in FIGURE 7-5 .

- When approaching the intersection, change the siren pattern from wail to yelp and use a short burst on the air horn before approaching the intersection.
- Continuously scan the intersection in all directions and monitor radio traffic for other assignment locations in case any other emergency vehicles are approaching the same intersection.
- Proceed slowly through the intersection. If there is other traffic waiting at the light, stop parallel to the rear bumper of the first vehicle in the left lane before proceeding. (STEP 1)
- Come to complete stop at the limit line. Wait for drivers to identify you, making eye contact with the drivers if possible. Watch vehicle wheel and driver head movement to confirm that drivers are slowing and stopping, and give your siren time to travel to other motorists and pedestrians near the intersection. (STEP 2)
- Next, pull up to the entrance of the intersection and wait for traffic to yield. (STEP 3)
- Continue with the siren in yelp and with short bursts of the air horn, as you pull up to the line that denotes

the next lane of cross traffic. Do not pass this line until you ensure that the drivers in that lane identify you and yield the right-of-way. (STEP 4)
- Clear each lane of traffic in this manner until you clear the intersection. (STEP 5)
- As you approach the center of the intersection, pay attention to traffic coming from your right that may not be able to see you.
- Do not stop scanning the intersection until you are completely through the intersection and traveling in your designated travel lane.

Intersections have many possible hazards, including objects such as buildings, trees, overgrown bushes, fences, billboards, or signs that could cause blind spots obstructing your view. Blind spots can also be encountered when traveling beside other vehicles. To ensure that you are not in another vehicle's blind spot, position your vehicle so that you can see the other driver's face in his or her side mirror. If this is not possible (e.g., tinted windows or nighttime driving), then position your vehicle so that your front bumper is parallel to or slightly further back from the other vehicle's rear bumper FIGURE 7-6 . In this position, the other driver should be able to identify you in his or her mirror. If you have sufficient room, you may also pull up, positioning your front bumper parallel to the other vehicle's side mirror so that the other driver can see you by looking out the driver's window. Other large vehicles may create moving blind spots, hiding smaller vehicles FIGURE 7-7 . If the hidden vehicle accelerates, it may not become visible until the point of impact. To avoid this situation, slow down to increase your view of the situation and the amount of time you have to react to a hazard.

Patient Transport

As an emergency vehicle operator, you will be asked to determine the need for emergency transport for patients in critical condition. You have probably seen countless movies and television shows where patients are whisked off in an ambulance with lights flashing and siren screaming. That makes for good television, but not good reality. The reality is that many patients will not need expedited transport to the hospital with lights and siren, and those who do will most likely not need to travel at a speed greater than the posted speed limit.

Transport of noncritical or nonurgent patients comprises almost 80% of EMS assignments according to a 2009 study. These patients are brought to the hospital with minimal out-of-hospital interventions and will most likely be triaged at the hospital and wait for treatment. EMS crews may try justifying rushing to the hospital, claiming that speeding will save the patient's life and get the unit back into service sooner. But the truth is that treating nonurgent calls as emergencies places you, your partner, your patient, and other motorists in danger. The proper way to transport noncritical patients is to follow proper protocols: securing the patient to the stretch-

STEP 1 Stop parallel to the rear bumper of the first vehicle in the left lane before proceeding.

STEP 2 Come to a complete stop at the limit line and wait for drivers to identify you.

STEP 3 Pull up to the entrance of the intersection and wait for traffic to yield.

STEP 4 Pull up to the line that marks the next lane of cross traffic and wait for traffic to yield.

STEP 5 Clear each lane of traffic one at a time until you are through the intersection.

Figure 7-5 Crossing an intersection against a red light.

Courtesy of FAAC, Inc.

OPERATOR INCIDENT

Many intersection crashes occur every year, some with disastrous consequences, as we have seen in previous scenarios. In 2007, an ambulance in Eliot, Maine, was traveling through an intersection with lights and siren engaged when it collided with a pickup truck. While no injuries were reported, the ambulance needed to be towed and incurred $4,500 in repair costs. Two additional ambulances were needed to respond to the original call and this collision. In 2008 in Portland, Oregon, an ambulance driving with lights and siren engaged crashed into two vehicles at an intersection. Two people were injured and needed to be transported to the hospital. The emergency vehicle operator was fined for failing to ensure that the intersection was clear. In 2009 in Tulsa, Oklahoma, an ambulance traveling with lights and siren engaged collided with a car in an intersection. Again, two additional ambulances were needed for this collision and another for the original assignment. While none of these collisions ended in death or serious injury, they still created a significant disruption of EMS service. Even though most ambulance collisions thankfully do not result in serious injuries or death, they are still very costly to the service and often to the individuals involved. And last but not least, they delay response and timely care for the patient(s) involved in the original call.

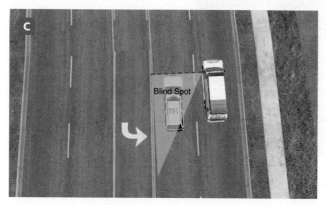

Figure 7-6 A. Do not position yourself between another vehicle's rear bumper and side mirror; this area is often in the driver's blind spot. **B.** Positioning your front bumper parallel to the other vehicle's rear bumper allows the other driver to see you in his or her side mirror. **C.** Parallel to the other vehicle's side mirror is also safe. When the driver looks out the window or at the side mirror, he or she will see your vehicle.
Courtesy of FAAC, Inc.

er or squad bench, securing all of the equipment to the unit, restraining all crew and passengers, and proceeding without lights and siren, obeying all traffic regulations.

When a patient is in critical condition, it may be necessary to engage lights and siren and take advantage of traffic law exemptions. Always travel at a speed that will be safe for the

Figure 7-7 The white truck has created a moving blind spot, hiding the blue car so that it is outside of the emergency vehicle operator's field of vision.
Courtesy of FAAC, Inc.

SAFETY POINTER

Know your vehicle's blind spots. Many ambulances have blind spots along the sides and back and below the windows and hood. The side mirrors, mobile data terminals, and A-posts (the vertical posts on either side of the vehicle's windshield that connect the roof to the body) may also create blind spots **FIGURE 7-8**. Make sure to signal, look twice, and merge over a period of 10 seconds.

Figure 7-8 The vehicle operator does not see the convertible (red outline), which is in a blind spot created by the ambulance's side mirror.
Courtesy of Rob Raheb.

patient and crew. Remember that transporting this patient to the hospital for definitive medical care is not your first priority. As the emergency vehicle operator, your number one job is to ensure the safety of yourself and your crew. However, bear in mind that even in the rare cases in which urgent transport is needed, you will be saving on average only about 40 seconds. If these seconds come at the price of rough handling, the crew in the back will not be able to perform the necessary patient care. Note also that in these situations equipment may need to be utilized during transport and may not be secured. This poses a dangerous condition, as the equipment can become a projectile if the ambulance takes sudden evasive action, injuring the patient or crew. If possible, vehicles should be equipped with mounts so that monitors and other equipment can be secured in a functional position.

SAFETY POINTER

The effects of a vehicle's dynamics are more magnified in the back of the ambulance than in the driver's seat. A small change in direction can throw the crew around in the back.

WRAP-UP

Summary

- As an emergency vehicle operator, you will need to determine how to balance the need for safety and the need for speed in responding to emergency calls.
- Communicate effectively with dispatch to gather the necessary information.
- Select an appropriate and safe route, minimizing traffic law exemptions whenever possible.
- Use warning lights and sirens appropriately to alert motorists and pedestrians of your presence.
- On a bidirectional roadway, you can clear traffic most effectively by positioning your vehicle as close to the center line as possible.
- On a unidirectional roadway, it is best to be in the middle lane or center of the road.

- When moving left of center on a bidirectional road, take the necessary precautions to ensure the safety of the crew and the surrounding traffic.
- To clear an intersection, use your sirens, scan continuously, proceed with caution, and clear only one lane of traffic at a time.
- Position yourself carefully to avoid being in other drivers' blind spots, and be aware of your vehicle's blind spots.
- Remember that you need to provide a smooth, safe ride for the patients and that a few seconds saved in transport rarely make a difference in patients' outcomes.

Glossary

air horn A warning device that uses compressed air, which is either electronically or manually controlled, to emit a unidirectional, long-range, low-frequency warning sound.

blind spot An area that prevents the driver from seeing the path or presence of an object.

Federal Q A well-known and distinctive type of wail siren that is trademarked by Federal Signal Corporation.

high–low frequency siren A siren sound with a sharp, clipped beginning and ending that cycles through higher and lower frequencies.

low-frequency siren A proprietary siren that works in conjunction with the vehicle's existing siren by producing an extremely low frequency that can shake (rumble) nearby objects.

moving left of center A traffic law exemption in which the emergency vehicle crosses over a dividing line and travels in opposing traffic lanes.

omnidirectional A sound that travels in more than one direction and can cause confusion in identifying the location of the source.

phaser A proprietary siren with a unique ray gun sound.

unidirectional A sound that travels in one direction, aiding in identifying the location of the source.

wail An undulating siren sound that is effective in notifying other motorists of your presence.

yelp A siren sound that rises in pitch and has a short clip at the end, extremely effective for clearing intersections.

References

1. Blackwell, T. H., Kline, J. A., Willis, J., Hicks, M. (2009). Lack of association between prehospital response times and patient outcomes. *Prehospital Emergency Care, 13*, 444–450.

2. NewsOn6.com. (2009, March 12). Tulsa EMSA ambulance involved in wreck. *NewsOn6.com*. Retrieved from http://www.newson6.com/story/9994223/tulsa-emsa-ambulance-involved-in-wreck

CHAPTER 8

Crash Prevention

OBJECTIVES

8.1 Discuss the factors that contribute to ambulance crashes.

8.2 Discuss the importance of employing defensive driving techniques and having a safe driving attitude.

8.3 Describe how to respond to dangerous driving conditions, such as skidding, running off the road, and tire failure.

8.4 Outline considerations for how to position the vehicle in a safe location.

8.5 List helpful resources for reviewing crash investigation reports.

8.6 Identify safety technology and vehicle design elements that can help reduce the likelihood of a crash.

8.7 Discuss what to do when a collision occurs.

SCENARIO

At the emergency department, Mike noticed that there were several other units present and that he would have to fit the vehicle into a tight space between two other vehicles. He did not want to bother his partner Shelly to get out of the vehicle to assist or to look out the rear window, so he began to back the vehicle into the space to the right. Mike knew this was the worst angle, as he was reversing into his blind side, but he continued anyway. He thought he was proceeding safely and slowly, but when he impacted the ambulance behind him, the force was enough to cause his partner to fall. Shelly had been standing in the patient compartment and was placing equipment in the overhead compartment, and she fell and hit her head against the compartment door. As a result of the impact, Shelly had a small laceration to her forehead and a hematoma. A few butterfly bandages were required to close her wound, and Mike had to write an incident report.

The ambulance service investigated the incident and made several changes as a result. First, the service added language to their standard operating procedures (SOPs) requiring partners to serve as a spotter when backing the vehicle if doing so would not compromise patient care. At the time of the incident, the service was in the process of designing specifications for new ambulances, and they decided to include backup cameras on the units as well as a right-side camera to help eliminate blind spots. The service also revised its guidelines to include restraint systems for the attendant providing patient care.

1. Do you always use a spotter when possible? If not, why don't you?
2. Do cameras eliminate all blind spots?
3. What other technologies could be used to avoid collisions?

Ambulance Crashes: A Serious Problem

Unfortunately, ambulance crashes are relatively common, with approximately 10,000 crashes each year. The National Highway Traffic Safety Administration (NHTSA) Center for Statistics and Analysis found that from 1988 to 1997, the number of EMS deaths was 12.7 per 100,000 EMS workers—a number more than twice the average occupational fatality rate. From 1992 to 2011, there was an average of 4,500 ambulance crashes each year, of which an average of 29 crashes annually involved at least one fatality. These figures corresponded to an average of 33 ambulance crash fatalities each year. There are many factors that contribute to the prevalence of crashes, including:

- Driver error
- Lack of vehicle performance
- Inadequate vehicle maintenance
- Poor vehicle design
- Lack of proper safety restraints
- Insufficient operator training
- Operator fatigue and distraction
- Lack of knowledge of specific traffic laws pertaining to emergency vehicle operations
- Inadequate policies and procedures for vehicle operation

This chapter examines steps the vehicle operator can take to avoid crashes and describes how to respond to a collision if one occurs.

Practice Safe, Defensive Driving

The best ways to avoid a collision are to drive defensively and have a safe driving attitude. This means being even-tempered, using good judgment, not demanding the right-of-way, and being courteous. Following these five common-sense rules can help reduce the likelihood of a collision:

1. Be aware of local laws and regulations that govern emergency vehicle operation.
2. Stay alert and anticipate other drivers' actions by aiming high in steering (down the road at least 12 seconds ahead) and constantly scanning to recognize any hazards.
3. Maintain proper following distance and spatial distance around the vehicle.
4. Always have an escape route.
5. Make sure other drivers can see you; keep your headlights on and avoid other vehicles' blind spots.

SAFETY POINTER

Ambulances typically have longer stopping distances than smaller vehicles on the road. Know your vehicle and always maintain a proper following distance.

The emergency vehicle operator must always travel at a speed that is safe for the current driving conditions. Many studies have examined the time savings gained by speeding, and while the time savings may appear significant to responders, the difference is rarely clinically significant to patients. If you want to save time, drive at a safe speed along the most direct route and call ahead on the radio so the emergency department is prepared for your arrival.

Finally, to ensure safety, it is best to avoid multitasking whenever possible. During an emergency response, the vehicle operator may be driving the vehicle, checking cross traffic, and listening to the radio or answering radio traffic at the same time. The driver's focus should be on safe operation of the vehicle. It may be necessary to delay answering a radio call until an intersection is cleared or the workload is reduced. When possible, best practice is for the EMS provider who is not driving to handle the radio and respond to radio traffic to minimize distractions for the vehicle operator. The other EMS providers should also help clear the intersection, watch for hazards, and help navigate.

Respond to Dangerous Driving Conditions

Inclement weather and hazardous driving situations such as loose gravel and leaves in the road are practically impossible to avoid; simply put, EMS cannot take time off for bad weather or road construction. However, when possible, it is best to avoid conditions that could cause the vehicle to skid. The most common causes of skids are driving too fast for existing conditions, failing to anticipate traffic conditions, not understanding the operational characteristics of the vehicle, misusing brakes and braking devices, and failing to properly maintain the vehicle. Some vehicles may be equipped with antilock brakes and electronic stability control to help prevent skids. In the event of a skid, you should release the brakes, allow the tires to turn to regain traction, and direct the front wheels in the direction of the skid. This means turning the vehicle into the skid and slowing without slamming on either the brakes or the accelerator.

In some hazardous situations, the vehicle may start to run off the roadway. Steering an emergency vehicle off of the road can lead to a serious collision. With one wheel off the pavement, there is less traction and the driver is fooled into turning the wheel more than needed. The most common reaction is to quickly steer the vehicle back onto the roadway, but doing so may lead to a dangerous overcorrection in which the vehicle crosses over lane dividers. Instead, if you run off of the road, gently remove your foot from the accelerator and continue to drive the vehicle steadily along the same path. Do not apply the brakes heavily, as doing so may cause a skid and pull you farther off the road. Gradually slow down and while keeping a firm grip on the steering wheel, smoothly turn the steering wheel to reenter the lane when traffic conditions and speed are safe to do so.

It is better to strive for a slow recovery, even if the vehicle suffers minor damage as a result.

Failure of a tire, such as a blowout, should be handled in much the same way as a run-off. It is important not to hit the brakes; instead, slow to a stop and work your way to a safe place on the side of the road. The ability to steer may be greatly compromised depending on which tire is blown. Activate the appropriate warning devices to alert traffic that you are disabled on the side of the road.

Position the Vehicle in a Safe Location

Emergency vehicles should be positioned appropriately at the emergency scene based on their function and need. For example, at an automobile crash, fire protection takes a priority, so fire apparatus must be able to stretch hose lines; if a patient is entrapped, rescue equipment must be able to reach the affected vehicle. If the ambulance is the first emergency vehicle on scene, then it will have to block the scene and should be parked with the wheels turned away from the work zone in case it is struck from behind. When blocking the collision scene, the best practice is to use "lane +1" blocking FIGURE 8-1 . Once EMS providers are ready to load the patient or after additional units arrive, move the ambulance downstream so that the collision scene protects the crew from traffic during patient loading. If emergency vehicles are on scene, then the ambulance should park with direct access to and from the patient, without having to expose personnel to traffic.

Ambulances should be positioned safely in a protected area at the scene. Ensure that the patient loading area is not exposed to traffic. Because most ambulances are loaded from the rear and personnel commonly operate in this immediate area, it is

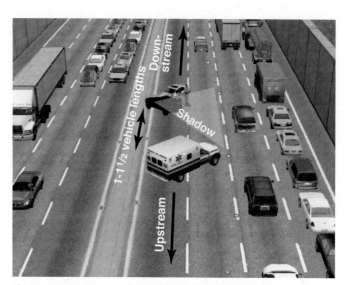

Figure 8-1 Proper ambulance positioning when it is first on the scene or is operating alone.
Courtesy of FAAC, Inc.

advisable to position the rear of the vehicle in a protected zone in front of the emergency scene, other rescue vehicles, and the flow of traffic. It is most effective to position the vehicle on the same side of the road as the incident if there is only partial road blockage so that personnel and preconnected hose lines are not required to cross or block lanes of traffic. Keeping one lane open will allow other emergency apparatus access into and out of the scene. On multilane roads, it is generally accepted practice to angle emergency vehicles away from the scene, in an effort to channel vehicles away from the scene, and to block additional lanes as needed to provide a safety cushion for emergency personnel on the scene.

It is also important to be cognizant of hazards encountered at private residences and in rural areas. Many homes have low hanging power lines or outbuildings with electrical supply that some ambulances may not be able to maneuver under. Septic systems in rural yards may also be hazardous, as trucks can sink into the soft ground above the septic tank.

When parking at scenes where ambulances may not be needed or other vehicles keep arriving, it is important to also consider egress. At fire scenes, additional working companies and hose lines can easily block ambulances in while they are on standby. At hazardous materials scenes, it is important to make sure the ambulance will stay in the cold zone (the area most removed from exposure and with the most readily available egress) even in the event of weather changes. Emergency vehicle operators need to be able to take patients to the hospital. If they do not consider the expansion of the scene and always have a way out, they will be unable to do their job.

SAFETY POINTER

Before leaving the scene, walk around the vehicle, making sure all equipment has been retrieved from the scene and secured and all doors are closed. This step also provides an opportunity to observe for any potential hazards.

Practice Safe Backing

Backing, or operating the vehicle in reverse, accounts for an estimated 25% of all emergency vehicle crashes. To help decrease the chance of a collision, a spotter should be used every time the emergency vehicle operates in reverse. The spotter should be positioned in a safe zone on the driver's side rear of the vehicle, and should be visible to the vehicle operator from his or her side mirror at all times. In situations where backing is necessary and a spotter is not available, the emergency vehicle operator should park the vehicle, get out, and assess the space available on all four sides of the vehicle prior to backing. Backup cameras, as well as alarms, are helpful but a camera should never be the emergency

vehicle operator's sole "eyes" on the situation. In addition to being a second set of eyes, the spotter is a physical deterrent to pedestrians and other motorists attempting to cross the ambulance's path. See Chapter 12 for considerations that agencies should follow when developing an emergency vehicle backing policy.

Learn from Other Crashes

One way agencies can reduce vehicle crashes is by researching and learning from past ambulance crashes. Several organizations publish crash investigation reports, including the following:

- National Institute for Occupational Safety and Health (NIOSH), www.cdc.gov/niosh
- National Highway Traffic Safety Administration (NHTSA) Fatality Analysis Reporting System (FARS), www-fars.nhtsa.dot.gov
- EMS Network, www.ems-network.com
- National Transportation Safety Board, www.ntsb.gov
- EMS Voluntary Event Notification Tool (E.V.E.N.T), event.clirems.org

Unlike the NIOSH program for fire fighter fatality reporting, no complete national incident reporting system exists for ambulance crashes, injuries, and deaths. The E.V.E.N.T. program is a voluntary EMS reporting system that EMS workers are encouraged to use to report incidents. By reviewing reports from these sources, an EMS service can help prevent the same mistakes from happening again.

Use Vehicle Safety Technology

Newer ambulances have been designed with technology to reduce the likelihood of a crash. External cameras provide better visibility for the driver and may include multiple camera heads, allowing the operator to choose between multiple views. Black box recorders monitor vehicle operational parameters and can be used to train vehicle operators, provide information for critiques, or help in investigations. Studies have shown that these technologies can reduce the likelihood of a collision and associated damage to the vehicle or injury to the occupants. Some of these technologies will signal drivers with sounds in the cab that they are doing something potentially dangerous while others may send real-time emails to supervisors, who can track trends in risky driving behavior.

Other vehicle design elements can increase safety as well. Adjustable seat placement and improved restraints protect attendants. Secure equipment storage can reduce risk of projectiles. (Note that cargo netting, although thought by many providers to reduce their likelihood of striking the bulkhead during a collision, has yet to be proven effective.) Turning and brake signal indicators in the patient compartment provide an attendant

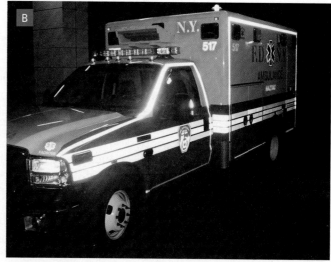

Figure 8-2 High-visibility paint on an emergency vehicle in **(A)** daylight and **(B)** at night.
Courtesy of Rob Raheb.

with visual warning of impending turns or stops. Changes in external graphics, high-visibility paint schemes, and LED lighting provide increased vehicle visibility. In addition, many manufacturers are now producing ambulances with curved and padded edges in the patient module for safety and convenience. Some are offering advanced airbag protection, along with three-point harnesses and head cushioning systems to protect attendants in the patient compartment. Seatbelt monitoring devices may be installed to alert the emergency vehicle operator if someone in the back is not properly restrained.

Some vehicles are equipped with traction stabilization controls. Traction control is a reverse form of antilock brakes. In situations where one wheel loses traction (such as on slippery surfaces), braking action is briefly applied to slow the wheel and help the vehicle regain control.

SAFETY POINTER

Even with advances in emergency vehicle design and technology, it is important to remember the most basic safety device—restraints. All occupants should be properly restrained, including those working in the patient compartment as well as any passengers and patients.

Vehicle Visibility Changes

Vehicle operators may be familiar with the *Manual on Uniform Traffic Control Devices* published by the Federal Highway Administration (FHWA) that defines the national standards for traffic control devices, road markings, and highway signs. This manual outlines requirements for temporary traffic controls, such as those needed when responding to a roadway incident. In addition, providers should be aware of the *Emergency Vehicle Visibility and Conspicuity Study* completed by the U.S. Fire Administration, which highlights best practices in emergency vehicle visibility to improve emergency vehicle and roadway operations safety. These practices include the use of retroreflective striping (a highly reflective substance that reflects light back to its source, with very little absorption or dispersion) and passive reflectors (which generally reflect light back at its source), called **chevrons**, and high-visibility paint for emergency response vehicles **FIGURE 8-2**. These design features are now used as a result of the study.

Crash and Near-Crash Events

If a crash occurs, it is important for providers to be familiar with state and local laws as well as the agency's SOPs. For example, many state and local laws require a motorist and vehicle involved in a collision to remain at the scene until police and/or other emergency vehicles arrive and permit them to leave. Agency SOPs may specify the following actions by the emergency vehicle operator:

- Report the incident via radio or per protocol
- Secure the scene to ensure safety until law enforcement or other responders can arrive
- Take care of any injured persons, including himself or herself
- Make no statements to anyone except law enforcement officers or your supervisors, until instructed to do so by and in the presence of legal counsel. This includes social media posts!

OPERATOR INCIDENT

As Tim arrived at the scene of the car crash, he took the only spot he could find—in the open lane across from the damaged car—and left the vehicle to attend to the patient. Tim and his partner had difficulty getting oriented. It was night time and a police car with flashing lights was parked facing their vehicle, making it difficult to see. Once they found the patient and were beginning to provide care, a crewmember from a second ambulance on the scene told Tim to move their vehicle, since they had the priority patient and the ambulance was blocking the road. Tim went to move the ambulance and realized he was blocked in. After some delay, he was able to move the vehicle across the street and return to the scene. When he got back, Tim's partner told him they would need immobilization equipment, so Tim had to cross back over the busy road to retrieve the equipment.

Tim realized as he crossed the busy road for a second time that he had not considered proper vehicle positioning on the scene, and later he sought help from his training officer. The training officer advised him to consider several factors before determining where to place the vehicle, including making sure the vehicle does not constitute a hazard on the scene or block traffic, ensuring equipment is available, avoiding contaminating the area with exhaust vapors, and ensuring that crew members are not unnecessarily exposed to traffic.

- Fill out required reporting documents
- Secure any equipment, such as narcotics and computers, if the unit will be towed and held for investigation

In addition, SOPs may indicate that supervisors should photograph the scene for reports. If the emergency vehicle operator is not a supervisor, he or she may need to discuss the need for photographs with his or her supervisor.

Companies should make sure employees receive any treatment and care before paperwork is done. Emergency vehicle operators should complete paperwork and incident reports as soon as possible while their memories are still fresh. All involved will probably have to give a statement and in many companies may have to submit to a drug and alcohol screening. These screenings, even if being done as required by policy, should be done hidden from public view.

Agencies may find it helpful to implement a **near-miss program**, which allows the organization to be aware of close calls that might otherwise go unrecognized. Most services have some procedure to review crashes in which their vehicles are involved. The intent of this review is to develop methodologies to identify patterns of dangerous behavior or procedures and provide the ability to share any information from lessons learned to prevent a recurrence. When this information is used to create updated protocols and policies, it may be helpful to ask the following questions:

1. Was a policy of the service violated?
2. Was the vehicle operator at fault?
3. Were there any mitigating factors (e.g., vehicle problem, equipment failure, road hazards)?
4. Has this situation occurred before? If so, what was done in the past?

WRAP-UP

Summary

- Defensive driving practices and a safe driving attitude are the keys to avoiding a collision.
- To ensure safety, avoid multitasking or driving too fast for road or weather conditions.
- If the vehicle skids, you should respond by releasing the brakes, allowing the tires to turn, and directing the front wheels in the direction of the skid.
- If the vehicle runs off the roadway, respond slowly to avoid a dangerous overcorrection.
- If a tire fails, slow to a stop and work your way to a safe place on the side of the road.

- It is important to determine the best vehicle position possible at an emergency scene to avoid hazards and ensure that all responders can function appropriately.
- A variety of agencies publish valuable reports on emergency vehicle crashes.
- Emergency vehicle design and safety technology can be used to reduce the likelihood of a collision.
- It is important to know state, local, and agency regulations for how to respond in the event of a collision.
- A near-miss program affords agencies the opportunity to learn from their mistakes.

Glossary

chevron An inverted V-shaped striping that slants downward at a 45-degree angle and reflects light; it is applied to the rear of emergency vehicles to increase visibility.

near-miss program A system that identifies situations that could have resulted in a collision in an effort to identify necessary revisions in procedures.

Additional Resources

Emergency Responder Safety Institute, www.respondersafety.com
EMS Network, www.ems-network.com
Manual on Uniform Traffic Control Devices (MUTCD), mutcd.fhwa.dot.gov
National Highway Traffic Safety Administration (NHTSA) Fatality Analysis Reporting System (FARS), www-fars.nhtsa.dot.gov

National Institute for Occupational Safety and Health (NIOSH), www.cdc.gov/niosh
National Transportation Safety Board, www.ntsb.gov

References

1. The National Highway Traffic Safety Administration, Office of Emergency Medical Services. (2014). *The National Highway Traffic Safety Administration and ground ambulance crashes*. Retrieved from https://www.naemt.org/Files/HealthSafety/2014%20NHTSA%20Ground%20Amublance%20Crash%20Data.pdf

2. U.S. Fire Administration, Federal Emergency Management Agency. (2009). *Emergency vehicle visibility and conspicuity study*. FEMA FA-323. Retrieved from https://www.usfa.fema.gov/downloads/pdf/publications/fa_323.pdf

CHAPTER 9

Driving Skills Course

OBJECTIVES

9.1 Describe and demonstrate the key components of an emergency vehicle operator skills course including:

- Physical requirements of the practice space
- Safety on the skills course
- Types of skill maneuvers

9.2 Describe and demonstrate the concepts of:

- Pretrip inspection
- Proper seat position for maximum control
- Proper hand placement on the steering wheel
- Key components in setting mirrors
- Proper mirror use
- Front-end depth perception
- Rear-end depth perception
- Left and right side judgment
- Off-tracking and turning

SCENARIO

You turn on the evening news and hear the following story: A 79-year-old woman in St. Paul, Minnesota, died after she was struck by a fire department ambulance that was backing down an alleyway to reach a patient. The victim was treated by paramedics and was pronounced dead at the scene. The mayor of St. Paul issued a written statement saying that words failed to express city officials' sadness for the woman's family and concern for the anguish of the paramedic crew. The city was undertaking an investigation to determine what happened and what changes need to be implemented to prevent this type of tragedy in the future.

1. What options other than backing are generally available when negotiating alleyways?
2. If this incident happened at your department, would standard operating procedures have been violated?
3. If you were involved in a situation such as this, how might it impact your personal and the department's reputation?

Introduction

It is important that all emergency vehicle operators being trained understand how a driving skills course is designed and the reasons behind this design. The driving skills course is an essential component of any successful vehicle operator training program. It is designed to help you understand the dynamics of the vehicle and its relationship to stationary objects around it. During skills training sessions, you will have a chance to perform maneuvers and make mistakes in a supervised setting. The skills course you will be using should ensure that the theoretical and didactic portions of the course are translated into competent and coordinated movement of the vehicle. You can study music and know everything about it, but until you actually pick up an instrument, you will never learn to play. The same can be said for driving an emergency vehicle well: You must get behind the wheel and gain hands-on experience. This chapter outlines the basic components that should be included in a driving skills course for emergency vehicle operators.

Setting for a Skills Course

Your instructor knows that the driving sessions should take place in an open area that is large enough to accommodate you and other students working and observing around the course but blocked off and protected from outside traffic. As you participate in a skills course, you will note that the area needed to perform a single maneuver is at least 10 times the vehicle's length and more than twice its turning radius in width **FIGURE 9-1** . In fact your skills course may be even larger, depending on which maneuvers you will be practicing on the range. Students should use the same vehicles they normally operate when possible. The course selected should have safety zones for observations, and there should be no permanent obstacles (e.g., utility poles) on

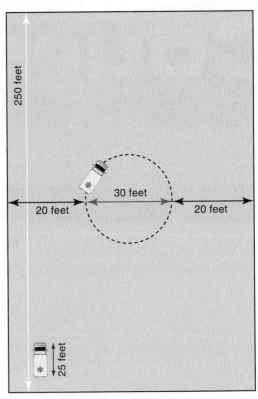

Figure 9-1 Practice space should have enough room for safe practice of maneuvers, including room to make mistakes and corrections.
© Jones & Bartlett Learning.

the driving course. Training sessions in the streets may be difficult at first and can lead to a series of problems, especially if the instructor has no control of the vehicle to override any dangerous mistakes. Courses may be physically arranged with stations to work on individual skills or as circuits in which several different types of maneuvers are connected in a series.

If the course is used for evening sessions, your instructor should select a location with proper lighting. Darkness can cause shadows and change the driver's perspective of distance so it is important to use light towers that are high enough to reduce shadows and bright enough to illuminate the field. Streetlamps or headlights do not provide sufficient lighting and may cast elongated shadows or blinding areas. Though not always possible, training at night can be very valuable to providers but proper lightening is required for everyone's safety. Recommendations for developing policies about safety on the driving range are discussed in Chapter 12.

Before Each Training Session

When beginning a training session, you should start by getting the vehicle ready by inspecting the vehicle and ensuring that the seat and mirrors are positioned properly.

Vehicle Inspection

The importance of vehicle inspection and maintenance for line units also applies to training units. Just as you will inspect your vehicle at the beginning of a work shift, you should plan to inspect the vehicle before starting any training sessions.

Seat Positioning

You will need to ensure that the seat is positioned properly before beginning the training session. The seat back should be positioned so you are sitting at a slightly reclined angle, 2 or 3 degrees less than 90 degrees; some students may find this position awkward, but it ensures maximum visibility and control. The seat is contoured so the body fits *into* it and not just against it, which helps to stabilize the driver during sudden changes in direction and acceleration. When the seat back is reclined too much, there is a gap between the seat back and the seatbelt, which can lead to excessive body movement, loss of control of the vehicle, and increased risk of injury.

The seat should be positioned so that you can reach both the accelerator and the brake pedal with your legs directly out in front, with a slight bend at the knee. The heel of the right foot should rest on the floor, able to depress both pedals without being lifted. Your chest should be a minimum of 10 inches from the steering wheel, allowing for airbag deployment, and your arms

should be close enough to the wheel to have a slight bend in the elbow when holding the wheel at the 9 o'clock and 3 o'clock positions. In this relaxed position, you can use all your upper body muscles if you need to turn the wheel rapidly. Sitting too close to the steering wheel diminishes the driver's range of motion and does not allow for total control of the vehicle. Additionally, if a collision were to occur, the relaxed position can help prevent serious extremity injury, which is more likely to occur when the arms are "locked" and straight.

Mirror Positioning

Mirrors must be positioned properly to help you know your relation to your surroundings. When adjusted properly, mirrors will provide a clear view of the road and help you avoid collisions **FIGURE 9-2**.

Wheel housing rubber molding

Driver's side mirror   Passenger's side mirror

Figure 9-2 Properly adjusted mirrors will ensure a clear view of the road.
© Jones & Bartlett Learning.

Figure 9-3 Look past the hood of your vehicle to get a clear view of the big picture.
© Jones & Bartlett Learning.

To correctly adjust the mirrors, you must first be sitting in the proper position. After the seat has been adjusted, sit with good posture to position the mirrors. Adjust the driver's side-view mirror so that the bottom two-thirds of the mirror are below the horizon, with a small sliver of the vehicle on the inside of the mirror and the top of the rear wheel housing in the bottom right (inside) corner. To adjust the passenger's side mirror, you should be able to see the top section of the rear wheel housing in the bottom left (inside) corner. In most cases, the passenger's side mirror is convex, which means objects in the mirror are actually closer than they appear.

Mirrors allow the driver to track the vehicle and keep it within the lane on a roadway. They also provide a line of sight to the sides for other obstacles that may block your movements. When driving in the skills course, you should be sure to use your mirrors in a continuous fashion. Scanning your mirrors every 10 seconds allows you to know what is to the sides of you so you can make safe, quick decisions. When turning, you should use both mirrors to ensure you have sufficient clearance. For example, when making a left-hand turn, you should use your left mirror to ensure that you do not sideswipe a vehicle or the center median, and you should use your right mirror to ensure that you do not impact a vehicle that may be trying to go around you.

Driving with Perspective

One of the most important aspects of the training course is its ability to help the vehicle operator become comfortable with the vehicle. Comfort with the vehicle requires knowing where the vehicle is in relation to other objects and roadway markers; thus the training course aims to develop the driver's perception of spatial relations.

To help develop a sense of front depth perception, you must first learn the distance between an object and the front of the vehicle. To do so, you should sit in the driver's seat and have an instructor or colleague drag a large cone (approximately 26 to 30 inches tall) toward the vehicle. When you can barely see the top of it, ask the person to stop. Repeat the exercise using a smaller cone (approximately 18 inches tall). Get out and look at the position of the cones in relation to the front of the vehicle. On average, the larger cone will be approximately 6 to 8 feet from the vehicle, and the smaller cone will be 10 to 12 feet from the vehicle **FIGURE 9-3**.

Similar judgment is used when backing to determine how far the vehicle can go without striking an object. This time, place a cone beside the rear of the vehicle and another at the farthest point at the rear of the vehicle (usually the step that can't be seen in the rearview mirror) **FIGURE 9-4**. You will need to know the full length of the vehicle, not just the box but also the extension of the rear step. If the vehicle has a backup camera, use the large and small cones to show the camera view in relation to the ambulance. This cone exercise will help you understand this spatial relationship between the two cones. With practice, you will be able to back the vehicle safely without striking any objects behind you. It is important to note that all backing should involve a spotter.

Side perception is also important because you will be required to maintain your vehicle in a restricted space, such as a lane of traffic, and position it in narrow spaces. The skills course can help you develop this ability through diminishing lane clearance and tight cornering drills. Drivers need to be aware of how far mirrors and steps stick out from the ambulance.

Turning the vehicle properly will require skills that address **off-tracking**. When a vehicle is traveling straight, the rear wheels should be aligned with (tracking) the front wheels. Off-tracking is what happens to the vehicle when the rear wheels are offset from the front wheels **FIGURE 9-5**. Off-tracking can happen for

Figure 9-4 Through understanding the spatial relationship between the two cones, you will be able to avoid backing into an object.
© Jones & Bartlett Learning.

Figure 9-5 All vehicles have off-tracking. The longer the wheel base, the wider the track, and the greater the angle that the front wheel can turn all play a part in off-tracking. The colored lines in each diagram demonstrate off-tracking—the purple line indicates the rear wheels and the green line indicates the front wheels. Notice how the rear wheels take a shorter path than the front wheels of each vehicle: **A.** Sedan. **B.** Type 1 ambulance. **C.** Conventional tractor trailer.
© Jones & Bartlett Learning.

several reasons that are problematic (e.g., a bent frame or poor wheel alignment), but it also happens routinely when the vehicle is turning. Failure to understand the amount of your vehicle's off-tracking could result in a sideswipe collision, so the skills course should include cornering and handling maneuvers to help you develop a sense of how off-tracking affects your vehicle.

The following factors affect the turning angle of a vehicle:

- **Wheel base** is the measure of the distance from the rear wheel hub to the front wheel hub. The longer the wheel base, the wider the track and the more of an angle the front wheel can turn.
- **Turning radius** indicates the width of the circle required for the vehicle to turn around without backing up. Take a circle and draw a line to its center: That is the radius. The tighter the turning radius, the wider the off-tracking will be.
- **Vehicle length** is the total length of the vehicle from bumper to bumper.
- **Wheel track** is the measure of the distance from the middle of the tread of the front tire to the middle of the tread of the other front tire; the sharper the angle the wheel can turn, the tighter the turning radius and the wider the off-tracking.

Table 9-1 **Common Skill Drills**	
Basic Maneuvers	**Advanced Maneuvers***
150-foot alley	Diminishing clearance
Serpentine (< 15 mph with cones 40 feet apart)	U-turn (left and right)
Lane change (15 mph at the decision point)	Switchback
Parallel parking (left and right)	Divider
Backing (left, right, and straight)	Evasive wall
Six-point turn (backing with spotter)	Skid control (if skid pad available)

*Performing advanced maneuvers may require a larger skills course, additional cones, greater vehicle speeds, and supervision by a more experienced instructor.

Skill Maneuvers

Once you have developed a sense of your vehicle and its relationship to your surroundings, you are ready to begin some skill maneuvers to develop vehicle control.

Your instructor should guide you through the sample common skill drills to help you practice skills such as coordinating and timing steering movements, maintaining proper hand position, judging the relationship of fixed objects to the vehicle, using mirrors appropriately, braking smoothly, and improving reaction time TABLE 9-1 .

These drills will give you practice developing vehicle directional control, including the ability to correct for off-tracking and negotiate the vehicle through narrow spaces.

For each maneuver, you may be asked to:

- Enter the maneuver at the required speed
- Keep the vehicle centered
- Check the mirrors
- Place the vehicle in reverse
- Carefully back out of the maneuver
- Control vehicle speed with the brake without bringing the vehicle to a stop until exiting the maneuver

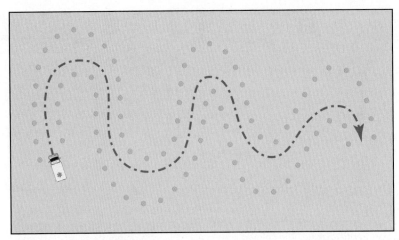

Figure 9-6   Be sure to allow for safety zones, mistakes, and corrections when performing the switchback maneuver. Turns in the maneuver need to be widened to accommodate vehicle off-tracking and front-end swing.
© Jones & Bartlett Learning.

You should receive instructions and a demonstration for each maneuver. To help build your competency and confidence, backing maneuvers on the skills course are typically performed without a spotter. A driver should never operate an emergency vehicle without a spotter in real-world conditions.

One example of a maneuver is the switchback. The **switchback maneuver** is a series of sweeping left and right turns that allows the student to develop left and right side judgment and front-end depth perception. The maneuver also teaches proper placement into the turn to allow for the off-tracking of the rear wheels without hitting cones with the front end, and it teaches matching of vehicle speed with steering wheel speed **FIGURE 9-6**. It is usually completed without brakes. Naturally, the faster you go, the harder it is to perform the maneuver, but it is important to remember this is not a race for completion. Safe, controllable speeds should be maintained at all times.

Your instructor will usually ask you to increase speed over several runs to (1) increase confidence and competency and (2) demonstrate that eventually there is a speed at which it becomes hard to control the ambulance. For example, imagine driving through a parking lot and turning the wheel all the way to the right and going through a turn; then, when partially through it, you must turn the wheel all the way to the left. The faster you are moving, the more skill will be required.

WRAP-UP

Summary

- The driving skills course is an essential component of any successful vehicle operator training program.
- Your instructor should design a skills course that has safety zones to allow for mistakes and corrections without colliding with any obstructions.
- When possible, students should use the vehicle or the same type of vehicle they regularly drive.
- Since multiple operators will be training on the same vehicle, it is important to emphasize vehicle inspection and proper seat and mirror adjustment prior to driving.

- The emergency vehicle operator should develop a level of comfort and experience with the factors that affect the turning angle of the emergency vehicle (i.e., wheel base, turning radius, vehicle length, and wheel track).
- All of the basic skills maneuvers should be practiced in a safe manner under close supervision by an experienced skills instructor and with a clear safety zone established during the maneuvers.

Glossary

off-tracking The offsetting of the rear wheels of the vehicle from the front wheels, as when the vehicle is turning.

switchback maneuver A series of sweeping left and right turns that allows the student to develop left and right side judgment and front-end depth perception.

turning radius The width of the circle required for a vehicle to turn around without backing up.

vehicle length The total bumper-to-bumper length of the vehicle.

wheel base The distance from the rear wheel hub to the front wheel hub.

wheel track The distance from the middle of the tread of one front tire to the middle of the tread of the other front tire.

Technological Aids

OBJECTIVES

10.1 Identify various technological aids that may be used in emergency response.

10.2 Explain how to use a global positioning system in emergency vehicle operations.

10.3 Outline how traffic preemption systems work to assist in emergency response.

10.4 Discuss how mobile data terminals can be used to assist in communication efforts.

10.5 Describe how driver behavior monitoring systems can be used to improve emergency vehicle operation.

10.6 Identify the benefits and potential hazards involved in using technological aids.

10.7 Discuss the value of new and future developments in EMS technology.

SCENARIO

Your ambulance is transporting an unstable 68-year-old female patient to the stroke center. You approach an intersection with a red light. As you enter the intersection, you slow down and begin to make eye contact with the other drivers. A car comes barreling into the intersection from your right. You do everything you can to brake and try to steer away, but the car hits your vehicle's rear right quarter panel. Your vehicle is turned onto its side. Both vehicles come to a stop in the intersection.

Your initial concern is for any possible injuries. Fortunately, everyone in your ambulance was wearing their safety restraints, including shoulder restraints on the patient, so no one was hurt. You inform the dispatcher of the need for police, the fire department, and additional ambulances to transport your stroke patient and to check on the other vehicle's occupants. You follow all the steps in your service's policy on what to do if involved in a crash. Your ambulance will be out of service until it can be repaired, and the car that struck you had significant damage to its front end. The vehicle's driver did not sustain any injuries.

The local media station ran the story on the evening news as the headliner, implying that you were at fault. Fortunately for you, the entire incident was recorded by a driver monitoring device that has been installed in your ambulance for the past two years. It shows that you were traveling at an appropriate speed, made eye contact with the other motorists in the intersection, and had attempted to navigate the intersection lane by lane when suddenly a driver using her cell phone went around the right of a line of stopped vehicles and ran right into the rear quarter panel of your vehicle.

1. How is technology improving ambulance and driving safety?
2. How is technology making emergency driving less safe?
3. In a perfect world, what technologies would you want your area to implement?

Introduction

Technological devices can be extremely useful in emergency vehicle operations. The modern technological aids discussed in this chapter are used to help emergency vehicle operators find the best route, preempt traffic lights, communicate with dispatch and other EMS providers, and monitor driver performance. As technology continues to develop, it will be the responsibility of your agency's management to evaluate new products and decide if they are cost effective and will help reduce the probability of crashes while making response safer for emergency vehicle operators, patients, providers, and the general public. It will be your responsibility as the emergency vehicle operator to be trained in and fully understand the operations of all technologies that become incorporated into the operation of the emergency vehicle.

However, technological devices are not perfect solutions. We will discuss the dangers of emergency vehicle operators becoming distracted by or over-reliant upon these devices. For example, just because your vehicle has an automatic backup alarm does not mean you do not have to be aware of who or what is behind the vehicle when backing up. Indeed many ambulances today have a camera to the rear of the vehicle, yet a small object or child could be missed if you are not careful and do not always use a spotter.

Global Positioning Systems

A **global positioning system (GPS)** device can be used to accurately identify an object's location. GPS was originally developed in the 1970s by the U.S. Department of Defense for locating ballistic missile submarines, and the same technology is now used to help locate many different objects, such as cellular phones and commercial and private vehicles. This technology relies upon 24 satellites orbiting the earth in precise locations and 5 ground stations that are used to triangulate the GPS device's location **FIGURE 10-1**.

In EMS, GPS technology has been combined with global system for mobile communications (GSM) wireless coverage to enable an agency to do the following:

-   Track an ambulance's location
-   Allow dispatchers to identify which vehicle is closest to an assignment location to reduce response times
-   Provide quick, efficient directions and rerouting
-   Save money by decreasing fuel costs
-   Use resources more efficiently

In some agencies without integrated GPS systems, personal navigation devices or smartphone applications may be used

A GPS satellite orbits and transmits a signal back to earth.

A vehicle's tracking device receives the satellites's signal, which determines the vehicle's location, speed, and direction of travel.

The tracking device transmits its position every 1–2 minutes through a cellular network.

Data is transmitted to an integrated server and relayed to the dispatcher, allowing him or her to select the closest vehicle to the assignment location.

Figure 10-1 A GPS device enables an EMS agency to track its vehicles and helps crews locate addresses efficiently.
© Jones & Bartlett Learning.

FIGURE 10-2 . There are some possible risks to using personal GPS devices for navigation. First, they may be a distraction to the emergency vehicle operator. Just as you should not be driving and reading the map, the GPS unit can be a distraction, moving your eyes away from the road and mirrors. If possible, your partner should serve as the navigator and guide you based on the GPS or map; this approach will allow you to keep your attention on the road. Typically the GPS programs in a smartphone involve a very small screen, and they can be a major distraction. Driving while using a cell phone may not even be legal in your state. It is your responsibility as the emergency vehicle operator to understand your state laws. If you have questions, ask police in your jurisdiction.

Figure 10-2 Personal GPS devices may be permitted by some agencies to assist with navigation. **(A)** Unmounted they are a distraction, and **(B)** mounted they are less distracting.
© Jones & Bartlett Learning.

> **SAFETY POINTER**
>
> Never attempt to program a GPS device while operating the vehicle.

GPS units, computers, and similar devices, depending on their placement in the vehicle, may block a section of the windshield and limit your view. When deciding to use a GPS

> **SAFETY POINTER**
>
> Always follow your agency's standard operating procedures (SOPs) regarding the use of GPS devices.

unit, seriously consider the policies of your service, the size of the GPS screen, and the location of the screen so that it does not interfere with your view of the road, traffic, and mirrors. It should also be easy to hear the directions over the other noises in the cab, such as the siren and communications radios.

Traffic Preemption Systems

Traffic preemption systems are a valuable technological aid to EMS response. These systems allow emergency responders to change traffic signals to allow them to clear an intersection and gain right-of-way. They rely on a series of receivers purchased by the municipality and installed at intersections with traffic lights, and emitters that are installed on the emergency vehicle **FIGURE 10-3** . When an emergency vehicle is responding to an assignment and approaches an intersection equipped with a traffic preemption system, the traffic light is preempted from its regular pattern. It will cycle through the caution (yellow) and red lights for all other directions, giving the green light and exclusive right-of-way to the

Figure 10-3 Traffic preemption systems work using infrared beams to trigger traffic lights to change, giving the emergency vehicle the exclusive right-of-way.
© Jones & Bartlett Learning.

emergency vehicle. This helps to clear the path in front of the emergency vehicle, which in turn can reduce response time. These systems can theoretically reduce the likelihood of collisions by giving the emergency vehicle the right-of-way, although their effectiveness depends on the volume of traffic and how long the emergency vehicle will be on the pathway being cleared by a series of green lights instead of the occasional red light.

Preemption priority is set so that if more than one emergency vehicle is approaching the intersection from different directions at the same time, only one will have the green light to proceed. Some systems include a flood light that notifies the public and other emergency vehicles of the direction of the emergency vehicle's approach as well as to confirm that the device has been activated. It is important to note that not all emergency vehicles are equipped with traffic preemption emitters. Therefore, it could happen that even if you have the right-of-way from your traffic preemption device, there could be another non-equipped vehicle attempting to proceed through the same intersection from a different direction. You should always use caution proceeding through the intersection, even with a traffic preemption device installed.

These devices can also be beneficial to patient care when they are used properly. Some services allow them to function independently of the emergency warning devices for transporting patients who are experiencing a time-critical event such as a stroke or heart attack. Using preemption devices allows the transporting ambulance to move efficiently through traffic but decreases the risk associated and the stress response the patient may have to emergency transport.

Mobile Data Terminals

Mobile data terminals (MDTs) are in-vehicle communication devices that have become the standard for many EMS agencies and emergency responders FIGURE 10-4 . Most MDTs are an extension of the computer-aided dispatch (CAD) system and extend the CAD capabilities. Some services utilize an in-vehicle laptop computer (mobile data computer, or MDC) that is mounted in the cab of the ambulance. These terminals or laptops can provide extensive response mapping, locate other units, and secure real-time access to public databases. MDTs increase information sharing and facilitate delivery of mission-critical information to the field (i.e., location of hazardous materials, building plans, and emergency plans). Many of the newer systems can provide electronic patient care report (e-PCR) capabilities and billing information, and can even be used for continuing education while the unit is posted at a location between calls. Some also use buttons to mark status changes to limit radio traffic, especially in larger systems.

MDTs are typically mounted in the cab between the seats on a swivel system, providing easy access to both the passenger and the emergency vehicle operator. Placement of the devices must not interfere with the vehicle's air bag system. MDTs should never be used by the emergency vehicle operator during vehicle operation, as doing so would distract the operator from driving duties. Also, depending on where they are mounted, they may create a blind spot or vision issues at night due to their bright screens. Always follow your agency's SOPs regarding MDT use.

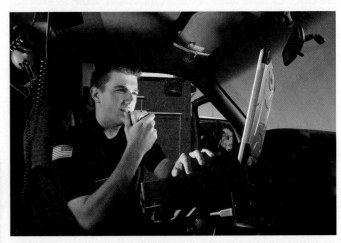

Figure 10-4 Mobile data terminals are a great resource for communication, planning, and reporting.
© Bounce/Cultura/Getty.

SAFETY POINTER

Traffic preemption systems are useful, but they do not remove your responsibility to ensure that the intersection is clear.

Driver Behavior Monitoring Systems

In the past, supervisors would have to accompany crews on the road to monitor driver performance or rely on observations and anecdotal evidence from other personnel to determine if emergency vehicle operators were using safe driving techniques. Unfortunately, this process of evaluation was inefficient, subjective, and unpredictable. Now, electronic driver monitoring devices can be used to monitor driver performance and help prevent collisions. These devices are also referred to as driver behavior monitoring systems (DBMS).

Driver monitoring devices record the driver's behavior, provide immediate feedback to the driver, and analyze the data to let the organization know the driver's overall compliance to driving standards. Electronic driver monitoring devices are valuable resources for evaluating and addressing any problems in driver performance. Using these monitoring devices, management may be able to determine which drivers need additional guidance and training before problems occur. In many cases, electronic monitoring can be used as evidence of a driver's innocence in the event of a collision.

Several different types of monitoring systems are available for EMS vehicles, including DriveCam™, envisionCAM™, Safety Vision™, and Road Safety™ FIGURE 10-5 . While there are some differences in how the specific devices work, the general concept is the same. They use data recording devices such as video cameras and/or sensors to record the vehicle's location, forward and lateral movement, and driver activities FIGURE 10-6 . In the event of any unexpected movement, such as a collision, quick acceleration, or sharp turn, the device will record information about the event, including use of turn signals, vehicle position and speed, and vehicle mechanical states (e.g., brake pressure). The data may be provided as real-time feedback to the driver and/or supervisors or may be analyzed by the manufacturer, with feedback later provided to the agency. The driver may be notified that an event has been recorded by a light on the device or an audible tone.

Management can review the recorded data with the emergency vehicle operator to provide further information or training regarding the event. Quality assurance personnel can maintain database files that track and cross-check different types of events, frequency of events, and event details such as certain

Figure 10-6 Monitoring devices can record drivers' actions.
© leaf/iStock/Getty.

time of day and weather conditions. Your service's driving instructor may share with members/employees in their emergency vehicle operator course some clips taken from these recording devices, noting specific lessons to learn from.

It is important to note that data from monitoring devices can serve as evidence to support the emergency vehicle operator in the event of a collision, and that the devices may also be used to provide safe drivers with positive feedback. Management can recognize personnel who are not involved in events that trigger the system and reward them for their safe driving habits FIGURE 10-7 .

These devices may be cost prohibitive for some services. Before implementing one of these types of system, administrators should check whether they can receive an insurance discount for these devices. It is believed that being monitored and recorded decreases bad driving habits, which can decrease collisions and costs to the insurance companies. Also, because the evidence can show that companies were operating safely, legal costs associated with liability issues may be decreased.

Figure 10-5 Sample driver behavior monitoring system.
© Safety Vision, LLC.

Figure 10-7 Rewarding personnel is one way to reinforce good driving habits.
© Jones & Bartlett Learning.

The Next Generation of EMS Technology

Since the new products in development are usually significant investments by the developing manufacturers, there is little "intel" on what devices are currently in development. One can only speculate that the systems in the ambulance will give us more computer-monitored feedback on the condition of the vehicle, its lights and compartments, and its handling. Just look at the advances in automobiles. There are guidance systems available in cars today that warn drivers when they are approaching danger and begin to slow their vehicle before a crash occurs. There are even systems that will parallel park an automobile! In the large trucks, adaptive cruise control will maintain a safe following distance behind the vehicle in front of the truck, and collision mitigation systems will slow the vehicle when there is danger of a collision.

More sophisticated GPS systems will be able to tell us where the traffic backups are and advise alternate routes to our calls. As health care moves to a paperless world, the use of e-PCRs and linkage to hospital patient data systems will become more prominent, eliminating duplication of documentation and arming the EMS provider in the field with historical data on the patient's medical record.

WRAP-UP

Summary

- Technology can be useful and improve response and safety, but it also has its limitations. Improvements such as backup cameras cannot replace an actual spotter.
- Global positioning system (GPS) units, mobile data terminals/computers (MDTs/MDCs), and other mapping devices have made responding easier, but they also can be distractions for the driver and should not be used when driving.
- Traffic preemption systems work to assist in emergency response by giving emergency vehicles the right-of-way at intersections.

- MDTs or MDCs can provide valuable run information on the location of and hazards involved in a call and can even track ambulances' status without use of the radio.
- Driver monitoring systems can give feedback to drivers and agencies that can be used to correct risky and dangerous behaviors as well as reward safe driving habits.
- Each new type of technology should be evaluated for both its potential benefits and its limitations.

Glossary

driver monitoring system A monitoring system that tracks driver actions, vehicle movement, and immediate environment around the vehicle using video cameras and sensors.

global positioning system (GPS) A satellite-based location and navigation system used to locate vehicles and provide directions to specific locations.

mobile data terminal (MDT) A computerized device similar to a laptop computer that is used to communicate with a central dispatch office.

traffic preemption system A system used to preempt traffic lights, giving emergency vehicles the right-of-way.

References

1. U.S. Department of Transportation, ITS Joint Program Office (2006). *Traffic signal preemption for emergency vehicles: a cross-cutting study.* FHWA-JPO-05-010. Retrieved from http://ntl.bts.gov/lib/jpodocs/repts_te/14097_files/14097.pdf

CHAPTER 11

Simulation Training

OBJECTIVES

11.1 Describe the value of simulation training in emergency vehicle operations.

11.2 Explain how a driving simulator can be used in emergency vehicle operator training.

11.3 Discuss how virtual worlds are used in simulator training.

SCENARIO

Miguel had just graduated from his EMT program. After several weeks of training, he was finally allowed to drive the ambulance. When a call came in for a cardiac patient in critical condition, he engaged the lights and siren and proceeded to the call carefully, clearing traffic along the way. As he approached a busy intersection, he tried to remember everything he was supposed to do. He remembered to pull left of center and proceed up to the intersection against the red light. He remembered to ease his way into the intersection, recognizing that the two lanes of traffic to his left had yielded the right-of-way. Miguel proceeded to the double yellow line and saw that the truck in the lane immediately to his right had stopped to yield the right-of-way as well.

Before his training, Miguel would have felt confident that this situation was safe and would have proceeded through the intersection, but during his simulation training, Miguel had encountered a very similar situation that caused him to now pause for a moment. The truck beside him was large and in a position to block his view of the second lane of traffic. He knew from simulation that there could be another vehicle approaching from the right that he could not see. So, he moved forward slowly, allowing his lights and siren to warn oncoming traffic and waited to be sure the intersection was truly clear before proceeding. When he pulled through the intersection, he saw the truck indeed had been concealing a smaller vehicle that had stopped, but easily could have sideswiped the ambulance if it had not heard the siren. In a simulation he could make a mistake, analyze the action, and change his behaviors so he would not make that potentially fatal mistake when out on the street. Miguel was grateful his simulation training had prepared him for this situation, and he proceeded safely through the intersection to the call.

1. Do you use simulation in driving training?
2. Typically, your first attempt at airway management and other such skills will be performed on simulators. Should the approach to driving skills be the same? Explain your reasoning.
3. Are there other aspects of EMS that are as risky as emergency driving?

Introduction

Emergency vehicle operation requires a foundation of solid basic driving skills and a clear understanding of vehicle and traffic dynamics. To achieve this goal, many EMS services are using simulators to provide an interactive learning environment where students can role-play in a realistic situation and learn from their mistakes. Simulation training allows emergency vehicle operators to synthesize the knowledge they have learned in their lectures, the motor skills they have developed in training, and the judgment they have acquired in their skills courses **FIGURE 11-1** .

With the help of technology, EMS agencies can now use simulation modules to replicate a series of complex events, just as the military, airline industry, and medical field have for their specialized training. Simulation allows students to gain "on the job" training in a supervised setting where no one gets hurt and no property is damaged. It is valuable training that helps emergency vehicle operators minimize collisions and maximize recognition and avoidance of hazards. In New York City, after services implemented driving simulation in their emergency vehicle operator training, intersection collisions decreased significantly. This reduction in crashes more than pays for the cost of the simulation equipment and the training program required.

Thanks to gaming systems such as X-Box™, Sony PlayStation™, Nintendo-DS™, and Wii™, today's young adults have been using simulation computer games since they were young children. They are very familiar with the hand–eye coordination it takes to play these games and are comfortable and quick learners in a simulated environment. Many of today's emergency vehicle operators have played driving games in the past. Some of the learning tools on the market today build on that knowledge base.

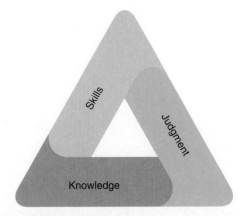

Figure 11-1 The triangle of training.
© Jones & Bartlett Learning.

Posit Science, which develops brain fitness programs, produced a gamelike computer exercise with the goal of improving reaction time, reducing crash risk, and increasing control in the majority of driving conditions. The American Automobile Association is promoting a program named DriveSharp, which has been shown to cut crash risk in half, improve stopping distance by up to 22 feet at 55 mph, and help older drivers maintain their driving skills as they age.

Driving Simulators

In a simulation training session, you will be practicing a realistic scenario using a **driving simulator**. Driving simulators are used in driver's education courses taught in educational training centers. They can also be used for research purposes to assess driver behavior and human factors. They present an opportunity for the student to experience road conditions, traffic conditions, and hazards and can even recreate actual collisions. Once the student gets behind the wheel of a simulator and receives some simple instructions in operating the "vehicle," the exercise can be challenging and fun at the same time.

Simulators used in EMS training are designed to mimic the department's regular emergency vehicles and should have full functionality (i.e., steering, gas, brakes, turning radius, stopping distance, and center of gravity of an actual EMS vehicle) **FIGURE 11-2**. One simulator can mimic several different types of vehicles. They may be open or enclosed cab units consisting of a driver's seat, dash console, steering wheel, pedals, siren, radio, and so on. The field of vision resembles a true driving environment, reflecting the view a driver would see through the windshield, windows, and mirrors, including blind spots. Driving simulators usually have a motion-based component that enables students to feel the inertia and dynamics of the vehicle **FIGURE 11-3**. The more realistic and closer to the handling and feel of the actual emergency vehicles that students will be using on the job, the less likely students will be to rationalize away performance as "only a function of using the simulator"; that is, they will be less likely to feel that their actions would be different if they were on the streets in their community in an actual emergency vehicle.

Your agency may send you to a training center for your simulation training or may arrange for mobile simulators at your site **FIGURE 11-4**.

SAFETY POINTER

Similar to how mannequins allow first-time EMS providers to safely practice clinical skills, simulators allow emergency vehicle operators to gain valuable driving experience without the consequences of real driving.

Figure 11-2 Fully enclosed simulators can mimic many different types of emergency vehicles.
Courtesy of FAAC, Inc.

Figure 11-3 Driving simulators on a motion-based platform can help provide training in vehicle dynamics.
Courtesy of FAAC, Inc.

Figure 11-4 Mobile simulators can be brought to your agency or training location.
Courtesy of Jack Armor and Three Rivers Community College.

Virtual Worlds

Similar to video games, simulations use **virtual worlds** in which emergency vehicle operators can practice new skills without repercussions. A virtual world takes the form of a computer-based simulated environment through which users can interact with one another and use and create objects. The term has become largely synonymous with interactive three-dimensional virtual environments, where the users take the form of avatars visible to others. Students are given freedom to choose which direction to go, how fast to go, and what to do. Most simulators will provide a variety of virtual worlds to mimic urban areas, congested streets, rural countryside, gravel roads, super highways, and so on **FIGURE 11-5**. In these virtual worlds, students can practice the skills they have learned, such as intersection analysis or soft shoulder recovery.

Many of these virtual worlds utilize geo-specific mapping technologies such as those used in global positioning system (GPS) mapping. The following technologies are fundamental to the creation of virtual worlds:

- A **geographic information system (GIS)** is a computer system that combines database management system functionality with location information. A GIS can capture, manage, integrate, manipulate, analyze, and display data that are spatially referenced to the earth's surface.
- **Geo-referencing** is the process of determining the location of data in physical space. This process often involves converting geographic data to a real-world coordinate system.
- *GPS* is a system based on satellites that allows a user with a receiver to determine precise coordinates for his or her location on the earth's surface. GPS mapping is a primary source of spatial data, that is, data that define a location.

Simulators can also mimic various weather situations so you can practice driving in rain, snow, fog, or bright sun to get used to situations with limited visibility. Within the virtual world, there may be ice or wind, and simulators can mimic these conditions as well. They can also present various traffic patterns so you can work on handling your vehicle in relationship to other motor vehicles, pedestrians, and/or animals running across the

Figure 11-5 Virtual worlds can be **(A)** rural, **(B)** suburban, or **(C)** urban driving environments.
Courtesy of FAAC, Inc.

road. Your instructor may join in your simulation, controlling various entities such as other motorists and interacting with you to work on specific skills or situations.

WRAP-UP

Summary

- Simulation training in emergency vehicle operations is valuable because it allows the emergency vehicle operator to experience the dangers and challenges of emergency driving without the consequences of real driving.
- Driving simulators can be used to teach most emergency maneuvers, mechanical failures, tire blowouts, and other

driving issues so that when they happen in the real world, it is not the first time the emergency vehicle operator is experiencing the situation.
- Virtual worlds are used in simulator training to create a realistic environment for emergency vehicle operators so they can react to real situations in a simulation.

Glossary

driving simulator A training tool used in driver's education courses to expose students to realistic driving situations and to assess driver behavior and human factors. Typically simulators involve a computer display of everything the operator would see through the windshield and mirrors during actual driving.

geographic information system (GIS) A computer system that combines database management system functionality with location information.

geo-referencing The process of determining the location of data in physical space.

virtual world A computer-based simulated environment through which users can interact with one another and use and create objects. The term has become largely synonymous with interactive three-dimensional virtual environments, where the users take the form of avatars visible to others.

References

1. Centers for Disease Control and Prevention. (2014). CDC - GIS (Geographic Information Systems). Retrieved from https://www.cdc.gov/gis/index.htm

CHAPTER 12

Standard Operating Procedures

OBJECTIVES

12.1 Explain the general process used to develop a standard operating procedure (SOP).

12.2 Describe the key concepts to incorporate in an SOP for backing the EMS vehicle.

12.3 Discuss the key concepts to incorporate in an SOP for the use of safety restraints.

12.4 Describe the key concepts to incorporate in an SOP for driving range safety.

12.5 Describe the key concepts to incorporate in an SOP for a crash involving an EMS vehicle.

12.6 Discuss the key concepts to incorporate in an SOP for visibility at the scene of an emergency call.

12.7 Describe the key concepts to incorporate in a sample SOP on qualifications for new emergency vehicle operators.

12.8 Describe the key concepts to incorporate in an SOP for the avoidance of distractions while driving.

12.9 Describe the key concepts to incorporate in an SOP for alcohol and drug use.

SCENARIO

You and your partner are dispatched to an unconscious patient on the opposite side of town, on a street with which neither of you is familiar. You race out of the station urgently, without checking the map, since your agency recently installed a new global positioning system (GPS) navigation device in your unit. It is late afternoon, the sky is clear, the sun is bright and shining, and the roads are dry. Once in the ambulance, you engage your lights and siren and start down Main Street. It is a two-way street with cars parallel parked on both sides, so you keep a lookout for pedestrians.

You now need to use the new GPS unit and reach over to turn it on. You have one hand on the wheel as you are entering the address into the GPS unit, when suddenly you look up at the road and notice the ambulance has veered about 2 feet to the right and is approaching a parked flatbed truck. You see it and apply the brakes, but it is too late.

The collision happens with such force that it tears off the right doors and sidewalls of the ambulance. The windshield breaks, shattering glass all over the front cab. Your partner is unconscious, and there is blood all over the inside of the front cab of the ambulance.

You shut off the motor of the ambulance and immediately call the dispatcher to request the police, reassignment of your original call to another unit, and an ambulance for your partner. You exit the vehicle and go over to care for your partner whose right arm appears to be severely torn from the shoulder and is bleeding profusely. You can hear sirens in the background from the approaching ambulance.

1. When new technology is introduced in your department, what type of training should take place?
2. Can a GPS or navigation system replace sound knowledge of your response zone and preplanning a route?
3. How accurate and efficient are GPS maps and routes?

Introduction

Each state has its own set of motor vehicle laws, and local municipalities and departments often have their own, more specific, regulations as well. In addition to these rules, an EMS agency should have its own guidelines, known as **standard operating procedures (SOPs)**. An SOP is a very specific guideline designed to clarify or enhance state and local laws as well as describe the step-by-step procedures that management expects all personnel to follow to safely accomplish a specific job. These policies in many cases will carry the weight of the law.

For example, state law may allow the driver of an emergency vehicle to be exempt from following the posted speed limit when operating an emergency vehicle during an emergency operation. The local law may have a posted speed limit of 30 mph. However, if the state does not limit the speed of an emergency vehicle during a response, then there is no cap on the rate of travel according to the state. Beyond expecting the emergency vehicle operators to take full responsibility for all of their actions, an agency may wish to create an SOP on this issue. Some agencies have developed SOPs designed to cap or limit the speed of their vehicles (i.e., no more than 20 mph over the posted speed limit). SOPs can be legally binding, and it is your responsibility to be familiar with your agency's SOPs and follow them. (See Chapter 3 for more on the legal considerations of SOPs.)

In this chapter we will discuss how SOPs are developed and their importance to every member of the organization. We will provide some key features of effective SOPs that every agency should seriously consider implementing if they do not already have an SOP on the specific topic.

SAFETY POINTER

Emergency vehicle operators must be compliant with the laws in their state and local jurisdictions as well as all agency SOPs.

How SOPs Are Developed

Since the emergency vehicle operator will need to follow SOPs in his or her agency, it is helpful to understand how they are developed. First there needs to be a topic or issue needing direction and/or clarification in which an SOP could be helpful. The officer, committee, or members who are empowered to develop the SOP should clearly define the problem or subject that needs to be addressed. (In our discussion here, we will pretend that you are the person charged with creating the new SOP.) Next, consider why the SOP is being developed and the need for its development. It takes time to develop a new policy, and it should not be an overreaction to an issue involving a single member or employee that could be better dealt with by meeting directly with the individual. Unfortunately, there are many policies in many organizations that were developed in this manner rather than dealing with the specific person who caused the problem. Remember, once it becomes the policy of your agency, everyone will need to become familiar with the SOP and follow it.

SAFETY POINTER

When developing a policy, you should first define the **SMART objectives** of the policy. The acronym SMART is used to describe the key characteristics of meaningful objectives: *s*pecific, *m*easureable, *a*chievable, *r*ealistic, and *t*ime-bound.

Next do some research on the topic. Usually a problem identified in your agency has been identified in other agencies, so it is helpful to ask around and see samples of how other organizations chose to resolve the issue. Obtain copies of other agencies' SOPs on the specific topic to see how they dealt with the problem. You are not bound to solve your agency's problems in the same manner as agencies that are different than yours. After defining the problem and analyzing the other available SOPs, it is time to write a first draft. It will be helpful to circulate the draft (clearly marked as "draft") to a representative group of your members and management to ask them for their feedback on the clarity of the SOP and suggestions for improvements. If your agency has a legal counsel, you should ask for input to make sure the new SOP does not violate any laws and will be enforceable. Most agencies have a numbering system for their SOPs so they can be easily indexed by subject and located in a manual quickly. The SOP should clearly state who it is issued by and the date it becomes effective.

It is always helpful to get the input of the members or employees so the final version of the SOP can have ownership, buy-in, and a commitment from them to learn and follow the new SOP. Take the time to issue all members or employees a copy of the SOP and provide training as needed. After an SOP has been implemented, consider a review of all SOPs on a regular (e.g., annual) basis to see if they are still relevant, warranted, and effective.

Be Familiar With Your Agency's SOPs

Emergency vehicle operators must learn and fully comply with their agencies' SOPs just as they are expected to follow the rules of the road. Some services have a limited number of SOPs, which they train in and have come to believe in as the accepted standard of behavior for their service. Other agencies have volumes of SOPs, which most of their members or employees do not remember. Since all will be held up to the policy should there be a legal action, it is best to have fewer policies that everyone fully understands and complies with. Just as all EMS providers have to learn and follow the treatment protocols, all emergency vehicle operators should be required to learn and follow the service's vehicle operation SOPs. If you must refer to a pocket guide version until you commit them to memory, then do it that way. At the very least, bring a copy with you to work and review them until you are familiar with them. Employers need to make sure the most updated SOPs are available to all personnel and that everyone receives updates if they are changed.

Recommendations for Policies

The remainder of this chapter provides recommendations to incorporate into the development of specific SOPs on the following topics:

- Backing of the emergency vehicle
- Seatbelts and restraints in the emergency vehicle
- Safety procedures on the driving range
- Post-collision guidelines
- Visibility at the scene
- Qualifications for new emergency vehicle operators
- Avoidance of distractions while driving
- Alcohol and drug use

Most of these recommendations come from SOPs that have already been developed and are in place in organizations across the United States today. Rather than including specific agencies' SOPs as models, since there are so many excellent ones available, we have highlighted the key concepts that should be addressed in each policy area.

Other topics your agency should consider developing into an SOP include the following:

- Use of emergency warning devices
- Parking and securing a vehicle
- Basic defensive driving
- Service animal transportation
- Nonemergency driving
- Emergency driving
- Education and training requirements for your service

Backing of the EMS Vehicle

It is estimated that 25% of all emergency vehicle crashes occur while the emergency vehicle is operating in reverse. The average emergency vehicle operator may travel thousands of miles going forward. This same emergency vehicle operator will back up only 1 or 2 miles per year. The ratio of time or miles spent driving in reverse to the percentage of collisions is very concerning. We have a serious problem when we shift into reverse. Therefore, considerations in developing a backing policy should include the following:

- Backing should be avoided whenever possible. Where backing is unavoidable, a spotter or an assistant outside the vehicle should be used even when backup cameras are present. Only emergency services personnel should be used to do this. If a patient is on board and a spotter is not outside, then the EMS member with the patient should get out and spot the vehicle, provided that he or she is not actively engaged in patient care.
- When placing the vehicle in reverse, the horn should be tapped twice to let your spotter and everyone else around know you are about to back up. In addition, the reverse alarm should be functional every time the vehicle is placed in reverse.
- If no qualified spotter is available, whenever possible, the emergency vehicle operator should park the vehicle, get out, and make a complete 360-degree survey of the space cushion around all four sides of the vehicle to locate any obstructions or hazards present before backing the emergency vehicle.
- Spotters are never permitted to ride the tailgates or running boards, or hang off the rear of any emergency vehicle in motion. Spotters should be located to the driver's side rear of the emergency vehicle in a safe position so they can be observed in the operator's mirror.
- Spotters should use the proper hand signals when the emergency vehicle is being backed. Uniform hand signals should be established as part of the backing policy. (Refer to Chapter 9 for images of sample hand signals.)
- The emergency vehicle should not be backed until the spotter is in the proper safe position and communicates via voice or visible signal to the operator. The spotter should always be visible to the emergency vehicle operator in the safe zone. If the emergency vehicle operator loses sight of the spotter, the vehicle should be stopped immediately. When the spotter is in the proper/safe position, the emergency vehicle can continue to back up.
- Backing should be done very slowly and with great caution. The vehicle's speed should be controlled with the brake and not the accelerator.

There are some general rules for the emergency vehicle operators and spotters to always consider when backing the vehicle:

- Never be in a rush when backing or parking.
- Do not start to back or park when unsure of the area.

- Do not put the emergency vehicle into reverse gear until it has come to a complete stop.
- When it is dark, use the side and rear spotlights when backing.
- If the emergency vehicle has a backup alarm and/or backup camera that can be disengaged, they should be in the on position at all times, especially when backing the emergency vehicle.
- When turning while backing, check front fender swing to avoid front-end collisions.

Finally, all emergency vehicle operators should practice backing the vehicle during their training. Start with backing between cones into a simulated garage. Try backing around the serpentine cone setup, and then practice backing into the garage at the EMS station.

Use of Seatbelts and Restraints

As EMS providers, we know better than the general public the traumatic and often fatal effects of automobile crashes. The life-saving impact of seatbelts and restraints has been well researched and proven by the National Highway Traffic Safety Administration. Most states have passed laws requiring drivers and the occupants of vehicles to be belted when the vehicle is in motion. Some states have included an emergency vehicle waiver in their seatbelt law.

In regard to the front compartment of an ambulance, there is no acceptable reason for the emergency vehicle operator to waive the seatbelt requirement. If a family member is allowed to ride along to the hospital, it should be the vehicle operator's responsibility to make sure the person is properly belted. If the individual refuses to wear a seatbelt, it is best to not allow him or her to ride in the ambulance, as the individual could be seriously injured if the ambulance should be involved in a collision.

SAFETY POINTER

To ensure that any friend or family member of the patient is safely restrained, the emergency vehicle operator should assist the individual in buckling up prior to driving to the hospital.

When there are EMS providers or any family members in the patient compartment of the ambulance and the vehicle is in motion, they should be seatbelted. Even though it is often legal for the crew to be unrestrained in the patient compartment, it is never recommended. Some would argue that it is not always possible to be belted in when providing care to the patient. In reality, this is a very rare occurrence, and the manufacturers of ambulances are working on developing seats in tracks that can restrain the EMS provider while providing care **FIGURE 12-1**.

Figure 12-1 Safety seat with full harness belting.
Courtesy of Bob Elling.

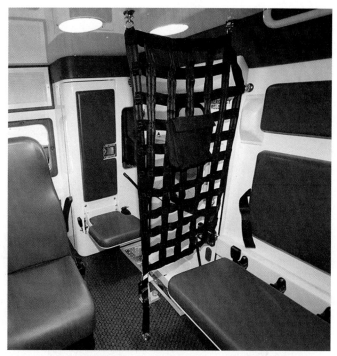

Figure 12-2 The cargo net is not an effective restraint device.
Courtesy of Crestline Coach Ltd.

Figure 12-3 A patient with shoulder straps properly applied.
© Jones & Bartlett Learning.

Many EMS providers believe that the cargo net hanging at the end of the bench seat is a restraint device. There are some who even refer to it as the "medic catcher," since they believe it will hang intact and protect the provider from coming off the bench seat and hitting the cabinets that are normally across the doorway from the bench seat. Some providers also use the cargo net as a storage device, from which to hang cleaning sprays, quick-access packs, stethoscopes, and other items. Hanging objects from the cargo net makes it unsafe as a restraint device, and its ability to hold a provider in place during a collision is doubtful since, as some collision videos depict, the force of the provider's impact can cause the netting to come free. The cargo net should neither be considered a restraint device nor used as a storage device **FIGURE 12-2**.

The patient should always be properly restrained in the seatbelts on the stretcher, including the over-the-shoulder restraint **FIGURE 12-3**. If a pediatric patient is transported in the ambulance, he or she should be restrained in a properly sized car seat or in appropriate strapping on the stretcher **FIGURE 12-4**. Car seats are not made or rated to be placed in lateral positions, such as on the bench seat or in the CPR seat; they need to be on the cot or in the airway seat (at the head of the stretcher). With an integrated child restraint system, the airway seat opens into a child safety seat, which can be used to transport a child who is uninjured or who does not require continuous and/or intensive medical monitoring and/or interventions **FIGURE 12-5**.

Safety on the Driving Range

When a skills course is set up to complement the didactic component of the emergency vehicle operator course, it is imperative that this exercise be treated as a potentially dangerous event and that all care is taken when one or more vehicles are on the driving range. Do not assume that any emergency vehicle operator, regardless of experience level, is watching the other students at the range. Exercises should be clearly explained and demonstrated by the driver trainer. The emergency vehicle operator should then be allowed to practice the specific exercise

Figure 12-4   An injured child should be transported in an appropriately sized child restraint system on the stretcher.
Courtesy of Evac+Chair International Ltd.

Figure 12-6   An EMS provider backing the ambulance on the range into some cones.
© Jones & Bartlett Learning.

Figure 12-5   An integrated child restraint system.
Courtesy of Serenity Safety Products.

(e.g., backing into a cone garage, serpentine maneuvers forward and backward, parallel parking the vehicle) without any other students on the driving range. It is not necessary to practice with a spotter in the backing exercises **FIGURE 12-6**.

There should be a clearly marked safety zone for other students in the class to stay within while awaiting their turn. Emergency vehicle operators who are driving the vehicles should stay away from the safety zones.

The training area should be large enough and free of obstacles to allow students to make mistakes without any consequences and without placing themselves or others in danger. As a rule, the range should be a minimum of 10 times the vehicle's length, and the width of the maneuver should include the total turning radius and the safe zone. The safe zone should be calculated as turning radius (TR) × ⅔ × 2. The purpose of multiplying by 2 is to account for each side of the maneuver. For example, if working with a vehicle that is 25 feet long, we would determine the minimum length of our field by multiplying 25 feet by 10, which is 250 feet. The proper minimum safe zone for a vehicle with a 30-foot turning radius would be calculated as 30 feet × .66 × 2, which is 40 feet (20 feet for each side of the maneuver). The total width of the training area would then be 70 feet (30 feet + 40 feet).

Procedures Following a Crash

Unfortunately, at some point, each service will experience an ambulance collision **FIGURE 12-7**. An emergency vehicle collision can present a major problem for an agency, but that problem can be greatly intensified if providers do not know how to regain control of the situation or are not aware of any plans

Figure 12-7   An ambulance crash scene.
© Larry McCormack/The Tennessean/AP Photo.

to deal with a collision. A policy for responding to crashes should include the following steps:

1. Notify the dispatcher right away and have the police, your supervisor, and other emergency services respond as necessary.
2. Determine whether there are injuries and whether an ambulance will be needed at the scene to treat and transport the injured, including your patient if you are carrying one.
3. Notify the dispatcher if the call you were responding to will require another unit to be sent in your place.
4. In most cases, it makes the most sense not to move the vehicles until the police have had the opportunity to document the scene. Moving the vehicles could have a detrimental effect on the investigation. Some states may have laws requiring vehicles to be moved out of traffic and not impede the traffic if there were no injuries involved. Follow your state and local laws as well as your department SOPs closely. If vehicles must be moved, take photos of the scene (not the damage) from a relative distance; try to include any road signs or markings and any geographic factors (e.g., hills, curves) that may have contributed to the collision. Also, mark the roadway at each point of the tires using the "T" method of a line alongside the tire and a line protruding out from the center hub. This helps in identifying the vehicles' positions.
5. Assign someone to deal with traffic appropriately until the police can take over that duty. Set up the proper flare or cone configuration that will assist motorists in identifying the collision and clearly move them away from the immediate area.
6. If the ambulance will need to be towed to a garage or body shop, make sure the drug box, HIPAA-protected documentation, and expensive equipment are removed and secured.
7. Services should have a policy that no personnel, except a designated public information officer, may talk to the media. Statements made while under duress could be inappropriate and come back at you or your service in a negative way.
8. If there is any injury, regardless of how minor, it should be evaluated at the time of the collision and not left until the following day. A worker's compensation package should be completed no matter how minuscule the injury.
9. All pertinent insurance information should be gathered as it would if the collision happened in a personal vehicle.
10. If law enforcement or department policies require a breathalyzer or field sobriety tests, make sure they are done out of the view of the public and news teams. Many times these are standard practices that can reflect poorly on the agency if shown in the media.

Visibility at the Scene

Traffic is a serious threat to the health and safety of the EMS providers and the emergency vehicle operator when working at the scene on a roadway. Whenever possible, law enforcement personnel will take responsibility for rerouting, stopping, or diverting traffic away from the EMS personnel and patients. All personnel must wear highly visible apparel, provided by the agency/department, when working in traffic on the roadway.

Qualifications for New Emergency Vehicle Operators

Your agency/department should clearly spell out what type of individual it is looking for as an applicant to become trained as an emergency vehicle operator. Considerations should include minimum age, years driving and clean record, maturity and good sense of responsibility, physical fitness, and dedication to improving driving skills.

The minimum duration and the specific objectives of the training program should be clearly spelled out. All emergency vehicle operator candidates need to understand the commitment they are making to become qualified.

It should be written in the SOP that the service will be conducting background checks of employees'/members' driver's licenses at the time of their initial application and/or qualification as an emergency vehicle operator as well as on a regular basis. It is the responsibility of the emergency vehicle operator to make the leadership of the agency aware of any serious infractions (points, moving violations, suspensions, crashes with injuries, DWIs/DWAIs) that occur while not at work at the agency. Many departments and states will require vehicle operators to carry their own automobile insurance even though they are covered by the department while working.

No Distractions While Driving Policy

Some states have already passed laws prohibiting talking on a cell phone and texting while driving because they take the driver's attention and hands away from vehicle operation. Yet, it is fairly common to drive down the highway and notice an emergency vehicle operator talking on a cell phone, talking on the radio, or in some instances texting or playing with the computer in the front of the ambulance. These are all distractions and can lead to a very serious crash. If you must use the phone, pull the vehicle over to a safe spot and use your cell phone to check in with your family or friends; do not do so while you are cruising down the highway.

As much as possible, eliminating the distractions to the emergency vehicle operator will help improve the safety of the ride to and from the call. Some services make it the responsibility of the crew member in the cab, who is not the driver, to deal with the radio transmissions and the maps or GPS devices while en route to the scene. Other distractions you may want to consider would include eating, drinking, and grooming while driving.

The bottom line here is that your SOP should be written in such a way as to minimize the distraction and create a sterile cab for the emergency vehicle operator.

Zero Tolerance for Alcohol and Drugs

The majority of the EMS and fire service agencies stand firmly behind EMS agencies strictly prohibiting any members or employees from responding to a call if they have been drinking. According to the International Association of Fire Chiefs' (IAFC) policy statement #3.04, Zero-Tolerance for Alcohol and Drinking in the Fire and Emergency Service (2003), "No member of a fire and emergency services agency/organization shall participate in any aspect of the organization and operation of the fire or emergency agency/organization under the influence of alcohol, including but not limited to any fire and emergency operations, fire-police, training, etc." The statement recommends that agencies develop written policies and have procedures in place for testing the blood alcohol levels of any individual involved in an incident that results in "measurable damage to apparatus or property, or injury/death of agency/organization personnel or civilians." The IAFC also suggests that any employee with an alcohol level of 0.02 or higher should be considered under the influence of alcohol. Both its 2003 policy statement and a subsequent position statement, "Drug and Alcohol-Free Awareness" (2012), recommend that members do not consume alcohol within eight hours of performing any emergency services duties. The 2012 position statement additionally recommends that agencies obtain legal advice and create policies that take into account the use of social halls for both department and non-department functions.

The IAFC's 2012 position statement also incorporates prescription and illicit drugs into its recommendations. Its position is that drug abuse should not be tolerated regardless of the type of drug, that there should also be zero tolerance of illegal drugs, and that agencies should have policies in place to test and suspend personnel during internal or external investigations. Prescription or over-the-counter drugs used while on duty should be approved by a healthcare professional and reported to a supervisor, who should verify that over-the-counter medications are allowed by the department physician and the safe use with the prescribing physician in the case of prescription drugs. The IAFC also suggests that Employee Assistance Programs be made available to members who are dealing with drug and alcohol abuse.

Each service's medical director, leadership and representatives from human resources, safety and risk department, and employee association or union should come to an agreement on a reasonable policy in reference to drugs, including prescription and over-the-counter medications, which can impair the emergency vehicle operator's driving abilities.

WRAP-UP

Summary

- Emergency vehicle operators must understand how and why agencies develop SOPs.
- Emergency services should develop a clear policy for backing the emergency vehicle.
- Emergency services should clearly define requirements for the use of seatbelts and restraints in the emergency vehicle.
- Safety precautions must be in place whenever driving skills are being practiced at the driving range.
- Emergency services should clearly state the specifics that emergency vehicle operators should follow if involved in a collision while operating the emergency vehicle.

- A department policy should exist in regard to visibility on the scene of an emergency call.
- Emergency services should clearly define the requirements for providers to become qualified as emergency vehicle operators.
- A clear policy should be in place for eliminating distractions to the emergency vehicle operator while operating the emergency vehicle.
- All EMS agencies must have a zero-tolerance policy in place for substances that affect emergency vehicle operators' coordination and judgment when operating an emergency vehicle.

Glossary

SMART objectives An acronym that describes the key characteristics of meaningful objectives: *s*pecific, *m*easureable, *a*chievable, *r*ealistic, and *t*ime-bound.

standard operating procedure (SOP) A policy issued by an agency's leadership to spell out how the employees or

members are expected to perform in a specific instance or circumstance.

zero tolerance A policy that makes a given behavior absolutely unacceptable; it does not allow for "three strikes and you're out."

References

1. International Association of Fire Chiefs. (n.d.). Guide to IAFC model policies and procedures for emergency vehicle safety. Retrieved from https://www.iafc.org/files/1SAFEhealthSHS/VehclSafety_IAFCpolAndProceds.pdf
2. International Association of Fire Chiefs. (2012). Position statement: drug and alcohol-free awareness. Retrieved from http://www.iafc.org/files/1ASSOC/IAFCposition_DrugAlcoholFree Awareness.pdf
3. International Association of Fire Chiefs. (2003). Zero-tolerance for alcohol and drinking in the fire and emergency service.

Policy Number 03.04. Retrieved from http://www.iafc.org/files/downloads/ABOUT/POLICY_STATES/IAFCpol_Alcohol_inFireEmergServ.pdf
4. U.S. Department of Transportation, National Highway Traffic Safety Administration (2012). Working group best-practice recommendations for the safe transportation of children in emergency ground ambulances. DOT HS 811 677. Retrieved from http://www.nhtsa.gov/staticfiles/nti/pdf/811677.pdf

GLOSSARY

4-5-12 rule A recommendation to maintain a 4-second interval between your vehicle and the vehicle ahead for speeds below 55 mph, increasing the following distance to 5 seconds for traveling speeds above 55 mph, and encompassing a 12-second visual lead time.

air brakes A braking system that uses air as a medium for applying the brakes.

air horn A warning device that uses compressed air, which is either electronically or manually controlled, to emit a unidirectional, long-range, low-frequency warning sound.

alternator An electromechanical device that converts mechanical energy to electrical energy in the form of alternating current; automotive alternators use a set of rectifiers to convert alternating current to direct current to charge the vehicle batteries.

antilock brakes A computerized braking system that prevents wheel lockup, helping the vehicle maintain directional control.

battery A device that chemically stores electrical energy; it is generally used for starting the vehicle and short-term electrical use.

black ice A thin film of water frozen on the road.

blind spot An area that prevents the driver from seeing the path or presence of an object.

brake fade A condition in which brakes become ineffective secondary to heat buildup in the braking system.

braking distance The physical stopping distance of the vehicle once the brakes are applied.

braking system The entire system that allows the vehicle operator to stop the vehicle by applying pressure to the vehicle's brake pedal.

camber The banking of the roadway; an arched road surface.

Centers for Disease Control and Prevention (CDC) The government agency that works to protect American health, safety, and security from all types of diseases, including those caused by human error and preventable problems.

chevron An inverted V-shaped striping that slants downward at a 45-degree angle and reflects light; it is applied to the rear of emergency vehicles to increase visibility.

civil law The type of law that pertains to determining responsibility for a wrongful act and imposing monetary penalties (with or without criminal charges) if the defendant is found guilty.

contour The curvature of a roadway.

criminal law The type of law that pertains to determining whether a statute has been violated and, if so, imposing a punishment (fine and/or imprisonment) on the guilty party.

crown The slope of a roadway, designed to facilitate drainage of water and debris.

defendant The person or party in a lawsuit who is charged with breaking the law and harming the plaintiff.

disc brakes A braking system designed with a disc and a brake caliper installed over the disc.

driver monitoring system A monitoring system that tracks driver actions, vehicle movement, and immediate environment around the vehicle using video cameras and sensors.

driving simulator A training tool used in driver's education courses to expose students to realistic driving situations and to assess driver behavior and human factors. Typically simulators involve a computer display of everything the operator would see through the windshield and mirrors during actual driving.

drum brakes A braking system that has a circular wheel hub with two semicircular brake shoes installed inside.

due regard Appropriate consideration and responsibility shown for the safety of others.

electrical system The system that generates and maintains electrical energy required for vehicle operation as well as for patient care activities.

Emergency Vehicle Operator Course (EVOC) A course launched in 1978 by the U.S. Department of Transportation to reduce the incidence of emergency vehicle collisions.

emergency vehicle operator The individual driving the emergency vehicle, generally an ambulance, who has the ability to operate it in the emergency mode (activating the lights and/or sirens).

engine A device that provides the mechanical motive force for propelling a vehicle and powering its subsystems.

exhaust system The system for removing dangerous exhaust gases from the engine.

Federal Q A well-known and distinctive type of wail siren that is trademarked by Federal Signal Corporation.

following distance The distance between a vehicle and the vehicle ahead of it.

friction Resistance of an object to slide over another.

geographic information system (GIS) A computer system that combines database management system functionality with location information.

geo-referencing The process of determining the location of data in physical space.

global positioning system (GPS) A satellite-based location and navigation system used to locate vehicles and provide directions to specific locations.

gravity A force that pulls objects toward the earth, resulting in what we know as weight.

gross negligence A more serious form of negligence that implies reckless conduct and a blatant disregard for the safety and lives of others. The line between negligence and gross negligence may need to be determined by a court.

gross vehicle weight rating (GVWR) The maximum allowable weight limit of a vehicle.

high–low frequency siren A siren sound with a sharp, clipped beginning and ending that cycles through higher and lower frequencies.

hydraulic brakes A braking system that uses fluid to charge and activate the brakes.

hydroplaning A driving situation in which a rolling tire rides up on a thin layer of water, preventing the tire tread from reaching the road surface.

inertia The resistance of an object to a change in its direction or speed.

inverter An electrical device that converts direct current to alternating current; it provides 110-volt current.

kinetic energy The energy of a moving object based on weight and speed.

liability Legal accountability or obligation.

low-frequency siren A proprietary siren that works in conjunction with the vehicle's existing siren by producing an extremely low frequency that can shake (rumble) nearby objects.

microsleeping A brief break with consciousness in which a person loses awareness of his or her surroundings and momentarily enters a state of sleep.

mobile data terminal (MDT) A computerized device similar to a laptop computer that is used to communicate with a central dispatch office.

morbidity Illness or harm; a diseased state.

mortality Death; the quality of being mortal.

moving left of center A traffic law exemption in which the emergency vehicle crosses over a dividing line and travels in opposing traffic lanes.

National Fire Protection Association (NFPA) A standards-setting entity that develops gold standards for the fire service.

National Highway Traffic Safety Administration (NHTSA) An agency of the U.S. Department of Transportation responsible for ensuring safe driving conditions.

near-miss program A system that identifies situations that could have resulted in a collision in an effort to identify necessary revisions in procedures.

negligence Failure to exercise due caution.

off-tracking The offsetting of the rear wheels of the vehicle from the front wheels, as when the vehicle is turning.

omnidirectional A sound that travels in more than one direction and can cause confusion in identifying the location of the source.

payload The total weight that a vehicle can carry within its gross vehicle weight rating.

perception distance The distance a vehicle travels during the time it takes to recognize a hazard.

phaser A proprietary siren with a unique ray gun sound.

plaintiff The person or party who files a complaint in a lawsuit claiming to have been harmed by the defendant.

potential energy The energy an object possesses while at rest.

preponderance of the evidence A requirement in determining the guilt of a defendant that the majority of evidence presented in a case favor the plaintiff's argument.

preventable collision A collision in which the driver failed to do everything reasonable to prevent its occurrence.

preventive maintenance Scheduled servicing, inspection, or replacement of specific items in the vehicle to reduce potential problems.

reaction distance The distance a vehicle travels during reaction time after perceiving a hazard but before applying the brakes.

reasonable doubt The lack of certainty that a person may justifiably feel based on the evidence at hand regarding the alleged guilt of a defendant.

road rage Aggressive or angry behavior by a driver of a motor vehicle that may include rude gestures, verbal insults or threats, or unsafe driving.

safety cushion An adequate vehicle clearance around all sides of the vehicle.

sipe A small slit in the tire tread that allows water to seep up within the tread block.

sleep deprivation The state of having an insufficient amount of sleep.

SMART objectives An acronym that describes the key characteristics of meaningful objectives: *s*pecific, *m*easureable, *a*chievable, *r*ealistic, and *t*ime-bound.

standard operating procedure (SOP) A policy issued by an agency's leadership to spell out how the employees or members are expected to perform in a specific instance or circumstance.

suspension system The system that supports the vehicle and allows it to absorb the impact from bumpy roads without affecting the ride inside the cab and patient compartment.

switchback maneuver A series of sweeping left and right turns that allows the student to develop left and right side judgment and front-end depth perception.

traffic preemption system A system used to preempt traffic lights, giving emergency vehicles the right-of-way.

transmission A device that provides speed and torque conversions from the engine to the wheels using gear ratios; it reduces the higher engine speed to the slower wheel speed, increasing torque in the process.

true emergency A situation in which there is a high probability of death or serious injury to an individual or of significant property loss.

turning radius The width of the circle required for a vehicle to turn around without backing up.

unidirectional A sound that travels in one direction, aiding in identifying the location of the source.

valve stem An opening to the valve that admits air to a tire and automatically closes to seal in pressure.

vehicle length The total bumper-to-bumper length of the vehicle.

virtual world A computer-based simulated environment through which users can interact with one another and use and create objects. The term has become largely synonymous with interactive three-dimensional virtual environments, where the users take the form of avatars visible to others.

wail An undulating siren sound that is effective in notifying other motorists of your presence.

wheel base The distance from the rear wheel hub to the front wheel hub.

wheel track The distance from the middle of the tread of one front tire to the middle of the tread of the other front tire.

yelp A siren sound that rises in pitch and has a short clip at the end, extremely effective for clearing intersections.

zero tolerance A policy that makes a given behavior absolutely unacceptable; it does not allow for "three strikes and you're out."

INDEX

Note: Page numbers followed by "*f*" and "*t*" refer to figure, and table respectively.